Mystic Christianity

Or, The Inner Teachings of the Master

William Walker Atkinson

Mystic Christianity; Or, The Inner Teachings of the Master

Copyright © 2021 Bibliotech Press
All rights reserved

The present edition is a reproduction of previous publication of this classic work. Minor typographical errors may have been corrected without note; however, for an authentic reading experience the spelling, punctuation, and capitalization have been retained from the original text.

ISBN: 978-1-63637-304-1

INDEX

LESSON
1.	The Coming of the Master	1
2.	The Mystery of the Virgin Birth	19
3.	The Mystic Youth of Jesus	36
4.	The Beginning of the Ministry	46
5.	The Foundation of the Work	58
6.	The Work of Organization	70
7.	The Beginning of the End	81
8.	The End of the Life Work	93
9.	The Inner Teachings	106
10.	The Secret Doctrine	118
11.	The Ancient Wisdom	132
12.	The Message of the Master	145

THE FIRST LESSON

THE COMING OF THE MASTER

THE FORERUNNER

Strange rumors reached the ears of the people of Jerusalem and the surrounding country. It was reported that a new prophet had appeared in the valley of the lower Jordan, and in the wilderness of Northern Judea, preaching startling doctrines. His teachings resembled those of the prophets of old, and his cry of "Repent! Repent ye! for the Kingdom of Heaven is at hand," awakened strange memories of the ancient teachers of the race, and caused the common people to gaze wonderingly at each other, and the ruling classes to frown and look serious, when the name of the new prophet was mentioned.

The man whom the common people called a prophet, and whom the exalted ones styled an impostor, was known as John the Baptist, and dwelt in the wilderness away from the accustomed haunts of men. He was clad in the rude garments of the roaming ascetics, his rough robe of camel's skin being held around his form by a coarse girdle of leather. His diet was frugal and elemental, consisting of the edible locust of the region, together with the wild honey stored by the bees of the wilderness.

In appearance John, whom men called "the Baptist," was tall, wiry, and rugged. His skin was tanned a dark brown by the winds and sun which beat upon it unheeded. His long black hair hung loosely around his shoulders, and was tossed like the mane of a lion when he spoke. His beard was rough and untrimmed. His eyes gleamed like glowing coals, and seemed to burn into the very soul of his hearers. His was the face of the religious enthusiastic with a Message for the world.

This wild prophet was most strenuous, and his teachings were couched in the most vigorous words. There was no tact, policy, or persuasion in his message. He hurled his verbal thunderbolts right into his crowd, the very force and earnestness emanating from him serving to charge his words with a vitality and magnetism which dashed itself into the crowd like a spark of electricity, knocking men from off their feet, and driving the Truth into them as if by a charge of a powerful explosive. He told them that the spiritual grain was to be gathered into the garners, while the chaff was to be consumed as if by a fiery furnace; that the axe was to be laid to the root of the trees which brought not forth good fruit. Verily, the "Day of Jehovah," long promised by the prophets, was near to hand to his hearers and followers.

John soon gathered to himself a following, the people flocking to him from all parts of the country, even from Galilee. His followers began to talk among themselves, asking whether indeed this man were not the long promised Master—the Messiah for whom all Israel had waited for centuries. This talk coming to the ears of the prophet, caused him to answer the question in his discourses, saying: "There cometh one mightier than I, after me, the latchet of whose shoes I am not worthy to stoop down and unloose; he that cometh after me is mightier than I." And thus it became gradually known to his following, and the strangers attending his meetings, that this John the Baptist, mighty preacher though he be, was but the herald of one much greater than he, who should follow—that he was the forerunner of the Master, according to the Oriental imagery which pictured the forerunner of the great dignitaries, running ahead of the chariot of his master, crying aloud to all people gathered on the road that they must make way for the approaching great man, shouting constantly, "Make ye a way! make ye a way for the Lord!" And accordingly there was a new wave of excitement among John's following, which spread rapidly to the surrounding country, at this promise of the coming of the Lord—the Master—perhaps even the Messiah of the Jews. And many more came unto John, and with him waited for the Coming of the Master.

This John the Baptist was born in the hill country of Judea, nearly thirty years before he appeared as a prophet. His father was of the priestly order, or temple caste, who had reached an advanced age, and who lived with his aged wife in retirement, away from the noise and confusion of the world, waiting the gradual approach of that which cometh to all men alike. Then there came to them a child of their old age, unexpected and unhoped for—coming as a mark of especial favor from God—a son, to whom they gave the name of Johanan, which in the Hebrew tongue means "Jehovah is gracious."

Reared in the home of his parents—the house of a priest—John saturated himself with all the Inner Teachings reserved for the few, and withheld from the masses. The Secrets of the Kaballah, that system of Hebrew Occultism and Mysticism in which the higher priests of Judea were well versed, were disclosed to him, and occult tradition has it that he was initiated into the Inner Circle of the Hebrew Mystics, composed of only priests of a certain grade, and their sons. John became an Occultist and a Mystic. When the boy reached the age of puberty, he departed from the home of his parents, and went into the wilderness, "looking to the East, from whence cometh all Light." In other words, he became an Ascetic, living in the wilderness, just as in India even to-day youths of the Brahmin or priestly class sometimes forsake their homes, renouncing their luxurious life, and fly to the jungle, where they wander about for years as ascetics, wearing a single garment, subsisting on the most elementary food, and developing their spiritual consciousness. John remained a recluse until he reached the age of about thirty years, when he emerged from the wilderness to preach the "Coming of the Lord," in obedience to the movings of the Spirit. Let us see where he was, and what he did, during the fifteen years of his life in the wilderness and hidden places of Judea.

The traditions of the Essenes, preserved among Occultists, state that while John was an ascetic he imbibed the teachings of that strange Occult Brotherhood known as the Essenes, and after having served his apprenticeship, was accepted into the order as an Initiate, and attained their higher degrees reserved only for those of developed spirituality and power. It is said that even when he was a mere boy he claimed and proved his right to be fully initiated into the Mysteries of the Order, and was believed to have been a reincarnation of one of the old Hebrew prophets.

THE ESSENES

The Essenes were an ancient Hebrew Occult Brotherhood, which had been in existence many hundred years before John's time. They had their headquarters on the Eastern shores of the Dead Sea, although their influence extended over all of Palestine, and their ascetic brothers were to be found in every wilderness. The requirements of the Order were very strict, and its rites and ceremonies were of the highest mystical and occult degree. The Neophyte was required to serve a preliminary apprenticeship of one year before being admitted to even partial recognition as a member and brother. A further apprenticeship of two more years was required before he was admitted to full membership, and extended the right hand of fellowship. Additional time was required for further advancement, and even time alone did not entitle the member to certain high degrees, the requirements being that actual knowledge, power and attainment must first be manifested. As in all true Occult Orders the candidate must "work out his own salvation," neither money nor influence having any weight.

Absolute obedience to the Rules of the Order; absolute

poverty of material possessions; absolute sexual continence—these were the conditions of membership to be observed by both Neophyte and Initiate, as well as High-degree Master. Understanding this, one may imagine the disgust inspired in John by the amorous solicitations of Salome, which caused him to lose his life rather than to break the vows of his Order, as is so startlingly pictured in the stage productions of modern times.

One of the ceremonies of the Essenes was that of Baptism (literally, "dipping in water") which was administered to Candidates, with appropriate solemnity and rites. The mystic significance of the ceremony which is understood by all members of Occult Orders, even unto this day, was a part of the ritual originated by the Essenes, and the rite itself was a distinctive feature of their Order. The performance of this rite by John the Baptist, in his ministry, and its subsequent acceptance by the Christian Church as a distinctive ceremonial, of which the "sprinkling of infants" of to-day is a reminder and substitute, forms a clear connecting link between the Essenes and Modern Christianity, and impresses the stamp of Mysticism and Occultism firmly upon the latter, as little as the general public may wish to admit it in their ignorant misunderstanding and materialistic tendencies.

The Essenes believed in, and taught the doctrine of Reincarnation; the Immanence of God; and many other Occult Truths, the traces of which appear constantly in the Christian Teachings, as we shall see as we progress with these lessons. Through its Exalted Brother, John the Baptist, the Order passed on its teaching to the early Christian Church, thus grafting itself permanently upon a new religious growth, newly appearing on the scene. And the transplanted branches are still there!

Of course, the true history of the real connection between the Essenes and Christianity is to be found only in the traditions of the Essenes and other ancient Mystic Orders, much of which has never been printed, but which has passed down from teacher to pupil over the centuries even unto this day, among Occult Fraternities. But in order to show the student that we are not making statements incapable of proof by evidence available to him, we would refer him to any standard work of reference on the subject. For instance, if he will consult the "New International Encyclopedia" (Vol. VII, page 217) article on "Essenes," he will read the following words:

> "It is an interesting question as to how much Christianity owes to Essenism. It would seem that there was room for definite contact between John the Baptist

and this Brotherhood. His time of preparation was spent in the wilderness near the Dead Sea; his preaching of righteousness toward God, and justice toward one's fellow men, was in agreement with Essenism; while his insistence on Baptism was in accord with the Essenic emphasis on lustrations."

The same article contains the statement that the Essenic Brotherhood taught a certain "view entertained regarding the origin, present state, and future destiny of the soul, which was held to be pre-existent, being entrapped in the body as in a prison," etc. (The above italics are our own.)

John emerged from the wilderness when he had reached the age of about thirty years, and began his ministry work, which extended for several years until his death at the hands of Herod. He gathered around him a large and enthusiastic following, beginning with the humbler classes and afterward embracing a number of higher social degree. He formed his more advanced followers into a band of disciples, with prescribed rules regarding fasting, worship, ceremonial, rites, etc., closely modeled upon those favored by the Essenes. This organization was continued until the time of John's death, when it merged with the followers of Jesus, and exerted a marked influence upon the early Christian church.

As we have stated, one of his principal requisites enjoined upon all of his followers, was that of "Baptism"—the Essenic rite, from which he derived his familiar appellation, "The Baptist." But, it must be remembered that to John this rite was a most sacred, mystic, symbolic ceremony, possessing a deep occult meaning unperceived by many of his converts who submitted themselves to it under the fervor of religious emotion, and who naïvely regarded it as some magical rite which "washed away sin" from their souls, as the dirt was washed from their bodies, a belief which seems to be still in favor with the multitude.

John worked diligently at his mission, and the "Baptists" or "Followers of Johanan," as they were called, increased rapidly. His meetings were events of great moment to thousands who had gathered from all Palestine to see and hear the prophet of the wilderness—the Essene who had emerged from his retirement. His meetings were often attended with startling occurrences, sudden conversions, visions, trances, etc., and many developed possession of unusual powers and faculties. But one day there was held a meeting destined to gain world-wide fame. This was the day when there came to John the Baptist the MASTER, of whose coming John had frequently foretold and promised. JESUS THE CHRIST appeared upon the scene and confronted his Forerunner.

The traditions have it that Jesus came unannounced to, and unrecognized by John and the populace. The Forerunner was in ignorance of the nature and degree of his guest and applicant for Baptism. Although the two were cousins, they had not met since childhood, and John did not at first recognize Jesus. The traditions of the Mystic Orders further state that Jesus then gave to John the various signs of the Occult Fraternities to which they both belonged, working from the common signs up until Jesus passed on to degrees to which John had not attained, although he was an eminent high-degree Essene. Whereupon John saw that the man before him was no common applicant for Baptism, but was, instead, a highest-degree Mystic Adept, and Occult Master—his superior in rank and unfoldment. John, perceiving this, remonstrated with Jesus, saying that it was not meet and proper, nor in accordance with the customs of the Brotherhoods, for the inferior to Baptize the superior. Of this event the New Testament takes note in these words: "But John forbade him, saying, I have need to be baptized of thee, and comest thou to me?" (Matt. 3:14.) But Jesus insisted that John perform the rite upon him upon the ground that He wished to go through the ceremonial in order to set His stamp of approval upon it, and to show that he considered himself as a man among men, come forth to live the life of men.

In both the occult traditions and the New Testament narrative, it is stated that a mystical occurrence ensued at the baptism, "the Spirit of God descending like a dove and lighting upon Him," and a voice from Heaven saying: "This is my beloved Son in whom I am well pleased."

And with these words the mission of John the Baptist, as "Forerunner of the Master," was fulfilled. The Master had appeared to take up his work.

THE MASTER

And, now, let us turn back the pages of the Book of Time, to a period about thirty years before the happening of the events above mentioned. Let us turn our gaze upon the events surrounding the birth of Jesus, in order that we may trace the Mystic and Occult forces at work from the beginning of Christianity. There are occurrences of the greatest importance embraced in these thirty years.

Let us begin the Mystic Narrative of Jesus the Christ, as it is told to the Neophyte of every Occult Order, by the Master Instructor, by a recital of an event preceding his birth by over one year.

In Matthew 2:1-2, the following is related:

> "Now when Jesus was born in Bethlehem of Judea, in the days of Herod the king, behold, there came Wise Men from the East to Jerusalem, saying, Where is he that is born King of the Jews? for we have seen his star in the East, and are come to worship him."

In these simple words is stated an event that, expressed in a much more extended narrative, forms an important part of the Esoteric Teachings of the Mystic Brotherhoods, and Occult Orders of the Orient, and which is also known to the members of the affiliated secret orders of the Western world. The story of THE MAGI is embedded in the traditions of the Oriental Mystics, and we shall here give you a brief outline of the story as it is told by Hierophant to Neophyte—by Guru to Chela.

To understand the story, you must know just who were these "Wise Men of the East"—The Magi. And this you shall now be taught.

THE MAGI, OR WISE MEN

The translators of the New Testament have translated the words naming these visitors from afar as "the Wise Men from the East," but in the original Greek, Matthew used the words "The Magi" as may be seen by reference to the original Greek versions, or the Revised Translation, which gives the Greek term in a foot-note. Any leading encyclopedia will corroborate this statement. The term "the Magi" was the exact statement of Matthew in the original Greek in which the Gospel was written, the term "the Wise Men" originating with the English translators. There is absolutely no dispute regarding this question among Biblical scholars, although the general public is not aware of the connection, nor do they identify the Wise Men with the Oriental Magians.

The word "Magi" comes to the English language direct from the Greek, which in turn acquired it by gradual steps from the Persian, Chaldean, Median, and Assyrian tongues. It means, literally, "wonder worker," and was applied to the members of the occult priestly orders of Persia, Media, and Chaldea, who were Mystic Adepts and Occult Masters. Ancient history is full of references to this body of men. They were the custodians of the world's occult knowledge for centuries, and the priceless treasures of the Inner Teachings held by the race to-day have come through the hands of these men—the Magi—who tended the sacred fires of Mysticism and kept The Flame burning. In thinking of their task, one is reminded of the words of Edward Carpenter, the poet, who sings: "Oh, let not the flame die out! Cherished age after age in its dark caverns, in its holy temples cherished. Fed by pure ministers of love—let not the flame die out."

The title of "Magi" was highly esteemed in those ancient days, but it fell into disrepute in the latter times owing to its growing use as an appellation of the practitioners of "Black Magic," or "evil wonder-workers" or sorcerers, of those days. But as a writer in the New International Encyclopedia (Vol. XII, page 674) has truly said:

"The term is employed in its true sense by Matthew (2:1) of the wise men who came from the East to Jerusalem to worship Christ. The significance of this event must be observed because the Messianic doctrine was an old and established one in Zoroastrianism."

The same article says of the Magi: "... they believed in a resurrection, a future life, and the advent of a savior."

To understand the nature of the Magi in connection with their occult "wonder working," we must turn to the dictionaries, where we will see that the word "Magic" is derived from the title "Magi;" the word "Magician" having been originally "Magian", which means "one of the Magi." Webster defines the word "Magic" as follows: "The hidden wisdom supposed to be possessed by the Magi; relating to the occult powers of nature; mastery of secret forces in nature", etc. So you may readily see that we are right in stating to you that these Wise Men—the Magi who came to worship the Christ-child, were in reality the representatives of the great Mystic Brotherhoods and Occult Orders of the Orient—Adepts, Masters, Hierophants! And thus do we find the Occult and Mystic "wonder workers"—the high-degree brethren of the Great Eastern Lodges of Mystic Occultism, appearing at the very beginning of the Story of Christianity, indicating their great interest in the mortal birth of the greater Master whose coming they had long waited—the Master of Masters! And all Occultists and Mystics find pleasure and just pride in the fact that the first recognition of the Divine Nature of this human child came from these Magi from the East—from the very Heart of the Mystic Inner Circles! To those so-called Christians to whom all that is connected with Mysticism and Occultism savors of the fiery sulphur and brimstone, we would call attention to this intimate early relation between The Musters and THE MASTER.

THE STAR IN THE EAST

But the Mystic story begins still further back than the visit of the Magi to Bethlehem. Did not the Magi say, "Where is He? We have seen His star in the East and have come to worship him." What is meant by the words, "We have seen his star in the East"?

To the majority of Christians the "Star of Bethlehem" means a great star that suddenly appeared in the heavens, like a great beacon light, and which miraculously guided the steps of the Magi, mile by mile, on their weary journey, until at last it rested in the heavens, stationary over the house in which the child Jesus lived, between the ages of one and two years. In other words, they believe that this star had constantly guided these skilled mystics, occultists and astrologers, in their journey from the far East, which occupied over a year, until it at last guided them to Bethlehem and then stopped stationary over the house of Joseph and Mary. Alas! that these vulgar traditions of the ignorant multitude should have served so long to obscure a beautiful mystic occurrence, and which by their utter improbability and unscientific nature should have caused thousands to sneer at the very true legend of the "Star of Bethlehem." It remains for the Mystic traditions to clear away the clouds of ignorance from this beautiful story, and to re-establish it in the minds of men as a natural and scientific occurrence.

This story of the "traveling star" arose from the superstitious and ignorant ideas of many of the Christians of the first, second, and third centuries after Christ's death. These tales were injected into the manuscripts left by the disciples, and soon began to be regarded as a part and portion of the authentic Gospels and Epistles, although the skilled Biblical critics and scholars of to-day are rapidly discarding many of these additions as wilful forgeries and interpolations. It must be remembered that the oldest manuscripts of the books of the New Testament are known to Biblical scholars to have been written not less than three hundred years after the time of the original writing, and are merely copies of copies of the originals, undoubtedly added to, altered, and adulterated by the writers through whose hands they had passed. This is not merely the statement of an outside critic—it is a fact that is clearly stated in the writings of the scholars in the Churches engaged in the work of Biblical study, and the Higher Criticism, to which works we refer any who may have reason to doubt our statement.

That portion of the verse (Matt. 2:9.) in which it is said that "and lo; the star which they saw in the east went before them, till it came and stood over where the young child was," is known to the Mystic and Occult Orders to be a rank interpolation into the story of the Magi. It is contrary to their own traditions and records, and is also contrary to reason and to scientific laws, and this distorted story alone has been the cause of the development of thousands of "infidels" who could not accept the tale.

All intelligent men know that a "star" is not a mere tiny point of flame in the dome which shuts us out from a Heaven on the other side of the blue shell, although this view was that of the ancient people, and many ignorant men and women to-day. Educated people know that a "star" is either a planet of our solar system, similar to the sister planet which we called the Earth, or else is a mighty sun, probably many times larger than our sun, countless millions of miles distant from our solar system. And they know that planets have their invariable orbits and courses, over which they travel, unceasingly, so true to their course that their movements may be foretold centuries ahead, or calculated for centuries back. And they know that even the great fixed stars, those distant suns and centers of great solar systems akin to our own, have their own places in the Universe, also their Universal relations and movements. All who have studied even the most elementary school book on astronomy know these things. And yet such people are asked to swallow whole this story of the "moving star," traveling on a little ahead of the shepherds for over a year, and at last standing right over the home of Jesus, and thus indicating that the search was ended. Let us compare this unscientific tale, with the traditions and legends of the Mystics, and then take your choice.

Had there been any such star in appearance, the historians of that day would surely have recorded it, for there were learned and wise men in the East in those days, and as astrology was a science closely studied, it would have been noted and passed on to posterity by both writings and tradition. But no such record or tradition is to be found among the Eastern peoples, or the records of the astrologers. But another record and tradition is preserved, as we shall see in a moment.

Yes, there really was a "Star of Bethlehem" which led the feet of the Magi to the home of the infant Jesus. We have the following proof of this fact:

(1) the traditions and teachings of the Mystic Orders which have been handed down from teacher to student for centuries;

(2) the statements and records of the Ancient

Astrologers, which may be proven by modern astronomical calculations; and

(3) the calculations made by modern astronomers, which shall be stated a few paragraphs further on. These three sources of information give us the same tale, as we shall see.

Before proceeding to a consideration of this three-fold evidence, let us pause for a moment and consider the relation of the Magi to Astrology. To understand the narrative of the Magi's Visit to Jesus, we must remember that they were the very Masters of Astrological Lore. Persia and the surrounding Oriental countries were the fountain-head of Astrological Teaching. And these Magi were Masters, and Adepts, and Hierophants, and consequently knew all that was known to the greatest schools of Astrology of that day. Much of their Ancient Astrological Lore has been lost to the race of to-day, but to these ancient learned men it was as much of a science as chemistry and astronomy are to the learned ones of our day.

The Magi had long waited for the appearance and incarnation of a Great Master of Masters, whose appearance had been predicted centuries before by some of the great Occult Fathers of the Mystic Orders, and each generation hoped that the event would come in his day. They had been taught that when the event took place, they would be informed by means of the planets, according to the Higher Astrology. All students of even our modern fragmentary astrology will understand this. And so they waited and carefully scanned the heavens for the sign.

Now the traditions of the Occult Orders inform us that at last the Magi witnessed a peculiar conjunction of planets; first, the conjunction of Saturn and Jupiter, in the Constellation of Pisces, the two planets being afterward joined by the planet Mars, the three planets in close relation of position, making a startling and unusual stellar display, and having a deep astrological significance. Now, the Constellation of Pisces, as all astrologers, ancient and modern, know, is the constellation governing the national existence of Judea. Seeing the predicted conjunction of the planets, occurring in the Constellation having to do with Judea (as well as the relative positions of the other planets, all of which played its part in the observation), the Magi knew two things, i.e., (1) that the birth of the Master of Masters had occurred; and (2) that He had been born in Judea, as indicated by the constellation in which the conjunction occurred. And, so, making the calculation of the exact moment of the conjunction, they started on their long journey toward Judea in search of the Master of Masters.

Now, again, the records of the Astrologers, preserved in the Oriental Occult Brotherhoods, in their monasteries, etc., show that at a period a few years before the Christian Era such a peculiar conjunction and combination of the planets occurred in the Constellation symbolizing the destinies of Judea, which was interpreted as indicating the appearance of an Incarnation or Avatar of a Great Divine Soul—a Master of Masters—a Mystic of Mystics. It must be remembered that these Orders are composed of non-Christians—people that the average Christian would call "heathens," and that therefore this testimony must be regarded as free from bias toward Christianity or the corroboration of its legends.

And, in the third place, the calculations of Modern Astronomy show without possibility of contradiction that in the Roman year 747 (or seven years before the Christian Era) the planets Saturn and Jupiter farmed a conjunction in the Constellation of Pisces, and that these two planets, still in close position to each other, were joined by the planet Mars in the Spring of 748. The great astronomer Kepler first made this calculation in the year 1604, and it has been since verified by modern calculations. To those who would object that all this occurred seven years before the commonly accepted date of the birth of Christ, we would say that any modern work on New Testament Chronology, or any encyclopedia or reference work on the subject, will show that the former calculations were several years out of the way, and that the records of other events mentioned in the Bible, such as the "enrollment" of the people, which brought Joseph and Mary to Bethlehem, enable modern Biblical scholars to fix the date of the birth of Christ at about six or seven years before the usually accepted time. So that modern research fully corroborates the astrological record and the Mystic traditions.

And so it would appear that the coming of the Wise Men—the Magi—was in accordance with the astrological signs, of the interpretation of which they were adepts and masters. When this truth is known, how puerile and petty seems the myth of the "traveling star" of the commonly accepted exoteric version? And the pictures of the Wise Men being led by a moving heavenly body, traveling across the skies and at last standing still over the cottage of Joseph, with which the Sunday school books are filled, must be relegated to the same waste-paper basket which contains the Bible illustrations, formerly so popular, which picture Jehovah as a bald-headed old man with a long white beard, clad in flowing robes designed to hide his body. Is it any wonder that skeptics, infidels, and scoffers of the spiritual truths have arisen in great numbers, when they have been asked to accept these things or be damned?

And is not this connection of Astrology with Early Christianity a rebuke to the modern Christian Church which sneers and scoffs at the science of astrology as a "base superstition" fit only for fools and ignoramuses? Does not this picture of the Magi give a clear view of that which was formerly regarded as a mere fable, to be solemnly smiled over and taught to the children, with whom the story has always been a favorite owing to their intuitive perception of an underlying truth. And now with this Mystic version, cannot you enjoy the legend with the children? In this connection let us once more quote from the New International Encyclopedia (Vol. II, 170), a standard reference work, as you know, which says:

> "Some of the earlier Christian Fathers argued against the doctrines of the earlier astrology, while others received them in a modified form; and indeed it formed a part of the basis of their religion in the Gospel narrative of the visit to Bethlehem of the Wise Men of the East, who were Chaldean Magi or Astrologers."

Here is the testimony in all of the standard reference books, and yet how many of you have known it?

To understand the importance of the event which drew the steps of the Magi to Bethlehem, we must realize that the Coming of the Master was a favorite subject of speculation and discussion among Occultists and Mystic organizations all over the Oriental countries. It had been foretold, in all tongues, that a Great Master would be given to the world—a mighty avatar or appearance of Deity in human form, who would incarnate in order to redeem the world from the materiality which threatened it. The Sacred Writings of India, Persia, Chaldea, Egypt, Media, Assyria, and other lands had foretold this event for many centuries, and all the mystics and occultists longed for the day "when the Master would appear." The Jews also had many traditions regarding the coming of a Messiah, who would be born of the seed of David, at Bethlehem, but their Messiah was looked upon as likely to be an earthly king, destined to free Israel from the Roman yoke. And so, the tradition of the Jews was regarded as of inferior moment to their own predictions, by the Mystic and Occult Brotherhoods of the East. To them it was to be an avatar of Deity—God in human form come to take his rightful seat as the Grand Master of the Universal Grand Lodge of Mystic—a descent of pure Spirit into matter. This conception certainly was very much higher than that of the Jews.

And so, knowing these things, we may readily understand why the Magi pursued their search with such ardor and enthusiasm. They had many weary miles of travel to Bethlehem, over a year being consumed in the journey. They reached Bethlehem over a year after the birth of Christ and the appearance of the Star, the sight of which had started them on their quest. They sought not a new-born babe, as common belief has it—they searched for a child born over a year before. (We refer the student to any reference work, for a verification of this last statement. The illustrations in the Sunday school books showing the Wise Men worshipping a new born babe in the manger are on a par with the others mentioned. The Wise Men had nothing to do with the stable or the manger—for Joseph, Mary and the Babe were lodged in a house by that time, as we shall see as we proceed.)

At last after their long and weary wandering over hill and plain, mountain and desert, the Magi found themselves in Jerusalem, inquiring diligently as to the whereabouts of the Master of Masters—the Promised One, whose coming had been the subject of prophecy for centuries among the Eastern peoples. The Jews of whom they inquired, although not familiar with the predictions regarding a Mystic Master, or avatar of Deity, were nevertheless thoroughly familiar with the prophecies of the coming of the Hebrew Messiah, and naturally thought that it was of this expected earthly King of the Jews that the Magi inquired, and so they reported it far and wide that these Great Men from the East had come to Jerusalem to find the Messiah—the King of the Jews, who was to deliver Israel from the Roman yoke. And, as the Gospel of Matthew (2:3) informs us: "When Herod the king heard it, he was troubled, and all Jerusalem with him." Naturally so, when it is remembered that it was an Earthly Kingdom that they expected the Messiah would inherit. And so, gathering the chief priests and scribes of Jerusalem around him, he bade them tell him the particulars regarding the prophecies regarding the Messiah—where he was expected to be born. And they answered him, saying: "In Bethlehem of Judea for so hath the prophets spoken."

And hearing the testimony of the scribes and priests, the wily Herod, who feared the realization of this old Hebrew prophecy which threatened to cost him his throne if fulfilled, called the Magi to his palace and in private consultation inquired of them the reason of their search. And when they told him of the astrological indications—of the "Star"—he was still more wrought up, and wished to locate the dangerous child. And so he inquired of them the exact date at which the star had appeared, that he might be better able to find the infant, knowing its date of birth in Bethlehem. (See Matthew 2:7.) And learning this he bade them go to Bethlehem and find the child they sought, and cunningly added, "And when ye have found him, bring me word, that I also may come and worship him." Thus craftily concealing his intentions to seize and kill the child, he endeavored to press the Magi into his service as detectives, by pretending to join in their desire to locate the Divine Child.

The Magi traveled on to Bethlehem, and arriving there made diligent inquiry regarding infants that had been born about the time that the star appeared. There were many infants born in Bethlehem during the same month, of course, and the search was difficult. But they soon heard strange rumors about a babe that had been born to travelers in Bethlehem about that time, the birth of whom had been attended by a strange occurrence. This peculiar happening is related in Luke 2:8-20, in which it is stated that at the time of the birth of Jesus in the manger, certain shepherds keeping the night-watch over their flocks saw an angel standing by them, and "the glory of the Lord" shining around about them. And the angel bade them be not afraid, for to them was to be given tidings of great joy, for there was born that very day, in Bethlehem, one who was to be the Anointed Lord of the world. And the angel further directed them that the babe would be found lying in a manger in a stable, wrapped in swaddling clothes which was to be their sign. And then suddenly the place was filled with a multitude of supernatural beings, praising God, singing, "Glory to God in the highest, and on earth peace and good-will among men." And the shepherds flocked to the town, and there found the child in the manger. And they spread abroad the report of the wonderful event accompanying the birth of the child. And consequently the child and its parents became objects of more or less public interest.

And so when the Magi instituted their search they were in due time informed of this strange occurrence. And they visited the house of Joseph and Mary and saw the Babe. Making close inquiry of the parents, they found that the time of the child's birth tallied precisely with the moment of the astrological signs. Then they cast the Child's horoscope and they knew that their shepherd's vision coincided with their own science, and that here indeed was He for whom the Eastern Occultists and Mystics had waited for centuries. They had found the Master! The Star Child was before them!

Then these Great Men of their own lands—these Adepts, Masters and Hierophants—prostrated themselves on the ground before the child and gave him the salutation due only to the great

Occult Master of Masters who was come to take his seat upon the Throne of the Grand Master of the Great Lodge. But the child knew naught of this, and merely smiled sweetly at these strange men in gorgeous foreign robes, and reached out his little hand toward them. But Occult tradition has it that the tiny fingers and thumb of his right hand, outstretched toward the Magi, unconsciously assumed the mystic symbol of the Occult Benediction, used by the Masters and Hierophants (and now used by the Pope in Papal Benediction) and gave to the worshippers that Master's benediction. The tiny Master of Masters thus gave his first blessing to his followers, and exalted worshippers. But His Throne was not that of the Great Lodge, but a still higher place—the knees of a Mother!

And the Magi then made mystic and symbolic offerings to the child—Gold, Frankincense and Myrrh offered they Him. Gold, signifying the tribute offered to a Ruler, was the first symbol. Then came Frankincense, the purest and rarest incense used by the Occult and Mystic Brotherhoods and Orders, in their ceremonies and rites, when they were contemplating the sacred symbol of the Absolute Master of the Universe—this Frankincense was their symbol of worship. Then, last symbol of all, was the Myrrh, which in the occult and mystic symbolism indicated the bitterness of mortal life, bitter though pungent, preserving though stinging—this was the meaning of the Myrrh, that this child, though Divine in his inner nature, was still mortal in body and brain, and must accept and experience the bitter tang of life. Myrrh, the strength of which preserves, and prevents decay, and yet which smarts, and tangs, and stings ever and ever—a worthy symbol of Mortal Life, surely. Wise Men, indeed, ye Magi! Gold, Frankincense, and Myrrh—a prophecy, symbol, and revelation of the Life of the Son of Man, with His indwelling Pure Spirit.

And the Magi, having performed their rites and ceremonies, departed from Bethlehem. But they did not forget the Child—they preserved a careful watch over his movements, until they saw him again. Saw Him again? you ask? Yes, saw him again! Though the Gospels say naught of this, and are silent for a period of many years in the Life of Jesus, yet the records and traditions of the Mystics of the East are filled with this esoteric knowledge of these missing years, as we shall see as we proceed. Left behind by the Magi, but still under their loving care, the Child waxed strong and grew in mind and body.

But the Magi, being warned by higher intelligences in a vision, did not return to the wily and crafty Herod, but "departed unto their own country another way." (Matt. 2:12.) And Herod waited in vain for their return, and finally discovering their escape wrathfully ordered the massacre of all male children that had been born in Bethlehem and its suburbs of two years of age and under. He calculated the two years from the witnessing of the "star" by the Magi. Matthew 2:16 states the story of the fixing of the time as follows:

> "And slew all the male children that were in Bethlehem, and all the borders thereof, from two years old and under, according to the time which he exactly learned of the wise men."

Herod sought to kill the feared Messiah—the King of the Jews, who threatened to drive him from his earthly throne—by killing all the male infants in Bethlehem that had been born since the astrological indication as stated by the Magi.

But this plot failed, for Joseph had been warned by "an angel in a dream" (which mystics teach was the Astral Form of one of the Magi) and was told to take the mother and child and flee into Egypt, and to stay there until the death of Herod. And so Joseph, Mary, and Jesus then fled from the wrath of Herod, and stole silently away to Egypt. And the Occult traditions have it that the expenses of the journey of this poor carpenter and his family—that journey into strange lands, hurried, and without the chance to earn money along the way—was accomplished by the means of the Gold that the Magi had offered to Jesus, and which they had insisted upon his parents storing away for His use. And so the gold of these Occult Mystics saved the founder of Christianity from massacre. And how poorly has Christianity repaid the debt, when one thinks of the persecutions of the Oriental "heathen" by the so-called Christians of all times!

And note this—they carried the child to Egypt, the home of Mystery and Occultism—the land of Isis! A worthy resting place for the Great Occult Master that was to be! And Occult tradition also has it that one night, wearied with their long journey, the family halted and passed the night in the place of the Sphinx and Pyramids. And that the Mother and Babe rested between the outstretched forepaws of the mighty Sphinx, which held them safe and secure, while Joseph threw himself on the base before them, and slept on guard. What a scene—the Master as an infant protected by the Sphinx, that ancient Occult emblem and symbol, while close by, reared like mighty watchful sentinels, stood the Great Pyramids of Egypt, the master work of Egypt's Mystics, every line and inch of which symbolizes an Occult Teaching. Verily, indeed is Christianity cradled in the lap of Mysticism.

Thus endeth our First Lesson. The Second Lesson will take up the Mystic Teachings regarding the Divine Incarnation of the Spirit in the mortal body of Jesus—a subject of the greatest importance to all who are troubled with this difficult point. We hope to be able to shed the Mystic light of Truth upon this corner which so many have found dark, non-understandable, and contrary to reason, natural law and science. The Mystic Teachings are the great Reconciler of Faith and Reason.

THE SECOND LESSON

THE MYSTERY OF THE VIRGIN BIRTH

One of the points of conflict between Established Theology on the one hand and what is known as Rationalism, the Higher Criticism, and Comparative Mythology, on the other hand, is what is known as "the Virgin Birth" of Jesus. Perhaps we may show the points of difference more clearly by simply stating the opposing views and, afterwards, giving the traditions of the Occult Brotherhoods and Societies on the subject. We are enabled to state the opposing views without prejudice, because we rest upon the Occult Teachings with a feeling of being above and outside of the theological strife raging between the two schools of Christian theologians. We trust that the reader will reserve his decision until the consideration of the matter in this lesson is completed. We think that it will be found that the Occult Teachings give the Key to the Mystery and furnish the Reconciliation between the opposing theological views which threaten to divide the churches into two camps, i.e., (1) the adherents of the established orthodox theology, and (2) the adherents of the views of the Rationalists and the Higher Critics.

The school of theology which clings to the old orthodox teachings regarding the Virgin Birth and which teachings are commonly accepted without question by the mass of church-goers, hold as follows:

> Mary, a young Jewish maiden, or virgin, was betrothed to Joseph, a carpenter of Nazareth in Galilee. Before her marriage, she was informed by an angelic vision that she would miraculously conceive a son, to whom she would give birth, and who would reign on the Throne of David and be called the Son of the Highest. This teaching is based solely upon certain statements contained in the Gospels of Matthew and Luke. Matthew's account is as follows:
>
> "Now, the birth of Jesus Christ was on this wise: When as his mother Mary was espoused to Joseph, before they came together, she was found with the child of the Holy Ghost. Then Joseph, her husband, being a just man, and not willing to make her a public example was minded to put her away privily. But while he thought on these

things, behold, the angel of the Lord appeared unto him in a dream, saying, Joseph, thou son of David, fear not to take unto thee Mary thy wife: for that which is conceived in her is of the Holy Ghost. And she shall bring forth a son, and thou shalt call his name JESUS, for he shall save his people from their sins. And now all this was done, that it might be fulfilled which was spoken of the Lord by the prophet, saying, Behold a virgin shall be with a child and shall bring forth a son, and they shall call his name Emmanuel, which being interpreted is, God with us. Then Joseph being raised from sleep did as the angel of the Lord had bidden him, and took unto him his wife: And knew her not until she had brought forth her firstborn son: and he called his name Jesus." (Matt. 1:18-25.)

Luke's account is as follows:

"And in the sixth month the angel Gabriel was sent from God unto a city of Galilee, named Nazareth, to a virgin espoused to a man whose name was Joseph, of the house of David; and the virgin's name was Mary. And the angel came in unto her and said, Hail, thou that art highly favored, the Lord is with thee: blessed art thou among women. And when she saw him she was troubled at his saying, and cast in her mind what manner of salutation this should be. And the angel said unto her, Fear not, Mary: for thou hast found favor with God. And, behold, thou shalt conceive in thy womb, and bring forth a son and shalt call his name JESUS. He shall be great, and shall be called the Son of the Highest; and the Lord God shall give unto him the throne of his father David. And he shall reign over the house of Jacob forever; and of his kingdom there shall be no end. Then said Mary unto the angel, How shall this be, seeing I know not a man? And the angel answered and said unto her, The Holy Ghost shall come upon thee, and the power of the Highest shall overshadow thee: therefore also that holy thing which shall be born of thee shall be called the Son of God." (Luke 1:26-33.)

And so, this then is the commonly accepted, orthodox teachings of Christian theology. It is embodied in the two best-known creeds of the church and is made an essential article of belief by the majority of the orthodox churches.

In the Apostle's Creed, which has been traced back to about the year A.D. 500, and which is claimed to have been based on an older creed, the doctrine is stated thusly: "... and in Jesus Christ, his only Son, our Lord, who was conceived by the Holy Ghost, born of the Virgin Mary," etc. In the Nicene Creed, which dates from A.D. 325, the doctrine is stated thusly: "... and in one Lord Jesus Christ, the only begotten Son of God, begotten of his Father ... and was incarnate by the Holy Ghost of the Virgin Mary," etc.

And so, the doctrine is plainly stated and firmly insisted upon by the orthodox churches of today, although such was not always the case for the matter was one which gave rise to much conflict and difference of opinion in the early centuries of the Church, the present view, however, overcoming those who opposed it, and finally becoming accepted as beyond doubt or question by the orthodox, believing Christian.

But the present time finds many leading minds in the churches, who refuse to accept the doctrine as usually taught, and the voice of the Higher Criticism is heard in the land in increasing volume and many doctrines unquestioningly held by the pews are being abandoned by the pulpits, usually in the way of "discreet silence" being maintained. But here and there courageous voices are heard stating plainly that which their reason and conscience impels. We shall now consider these dissenting opinions.

We have to say here, at this point, that we have no sympathy for the so-called "infidel" opinion, which holds that the whole tale of the Virgin Birth was invented to conceal the illegitimate birth of Jesus. Such a view is based neither on intelligent investigation or criticism, or upon the occult teachings. It was merely "invented" itself, by those who were unable to accept current theology and who, when driven from the churches, built up a crude system of reconstructed Biblical History of their own. And so we shall not stop to even consider this view of the matter, but shall pass on to the scholarly objectors and their views and thence to the Occult Teachings.

In the first place, the theologians who favor the views of the Higher Criticism object to the idea of the Virgin Birth upon several general grounds, among which the following are the principal ones:

> (1) That the story of the Divine Conception, that is the conception by a woman of a child without a human father, and by means of a miraculous act on the part of Deity, is one found among the traditions, legends and

beliefs of many heathen and pagan nations. Nearly all of the old Oriental religions, antedating Christianity by many centuries, contain stories of this kind concerning their gods, prophets and great leaders. The critics hold that the story of the Virgin Birth and Divine Conception were borrowed outright from these pagan legends and incorporated into the Christian Writings after the death of Christ;

(2) that the idea of the Virgin Birth was not an original Christian Doctrine, but was injected into the Teachings at a date about one hundred years, or nearly so, after the beginning of the Christian Era; this view being corroborated by the fact that the New Testament Writings themselves contain very little mention of the idea, the only mention of it being in two of the Gospels, those of St. Matthew and St. Luke—St. Mark and St. John containing no mention of the matter, which would not likely be the case had it been an accepted belief in the early days of Christianity—and no mention being made of it in the Epistles, even Paul being utterly silent on the question. They claim that the Virgin Birth was unknown to the primitive Christians and was not heard of until its "borrowing" from pagan beliefs many years after. In support of their idea, as above stated, they call attention to the fact that the New Testament writings, known to Biblical students as the oldest and earliest, make no mention of the idea; and that Paul ignores it completely, as well as the other writers;

(3) that the Gospels of St. Matthew and St. Luke bear internal evidences of the introduction of the story at a later date. This matter we shall now consider, from the point of view of the Higher Criticism within the body of the Church.

In the first place, let us consider the Gospel of St. Matthew. The majority of people accept this as having been written by St. Matthew, with his own hand, during his ministry; and that the Gospel, word for word, is the work of this great apostle. This idea, however, is not held for a moment by the educated clergy, as may be seen by a reference to any prominent theological work of late years, or even in the pages of a good encyclopedia. The investigators have made diligent researches concerning the probable authorship of the New Testament books and their reports would surprise many faithful church-goers who are not acquainted with the facts of the case. There is no warrant, outside of tradition and custom, for the belief that Matthew wrote the Gospel accredited to him, at least in its present shape. Without going deeply into the argument of the investigators (which may be found in any recent work on the History of the Gospels) we would say that the generally accepted conclusion now held by the authorities is that the Gospel commonly accredited to St. Matthew is the work of some unknown hand or hands, which was produced during the latter part of the first century A.D., written in Greek, and most likely an enlargement or elaboration of certain Aramaic writings entitled, "Sayings of Jesus," which are thought to have been written by Matthew himself. In other words, even the most conservative of the critics do not claim that the Gospel of St. Matthew is anything more than an enlargement, elaboration or development of Matthew's earlier writings, written many years before the elaboration of the present "Gospel." The more radical critics take an even less respectful view. This being the fact, it may be readily seen how easy it would have been for the latter-day "elaborator" to introduce the then current legend of the Virgin Birth, borrowed from pagan sources.

As a further internal evidence of such interpolation of outside matter, the critics point to the fact that while the Gospel of Matthew is made to claim that Joseph was merely the reputed father of the child of Mary, the same Gospel, in its very first chapter (Matt. 1) gives the genealogy of Jesus from David to Joseph the husband of Mary, in order to prove that Jesus came from the "House of David," in accordance with the Messianic tradition. The chapter begins with the words, "The book of the generation of Jesus Christ, the son of David, the son of Abraham" (Matt. 1), and then goes on to name fourteen generations from Abraham to David; fourteen generations from David to the days of the carrying away into Babylon; and fourteen generations from the Babylonian days until the birth of Jesus. The critics call attention to this recital of Jesus's descent, through Joseph, from the House of David, which is but one of the many indications that the original Matthew inclined quite strongly to the view that Jesus was the Hebrew Messiah, come to reign upon the throne of David, rather than a Divine Avatar or Incarnation.

The critics point to the fact that if Joseph were not the real father of Jesus, where would be the sense and purpose of proving his descent from David through Joseph? It is pertinently asked, "Why the necessity or purpose of the recital of Joseph's genealogy, as applied to Jesus, if indeed Jesus were not truly the son of

Joseph?" The explanation of the critics is that the earlier writings of Matthew contained nothing regarding the Virgin Birth, Matthew having heard nothing of this pagan legend, and that naturally he gave the genealogy of Jesus from David and Abraham. If one omits the verses 18-25 from Matthew's Gospel, he will see the logical relation of the genealogy to the rest of the account—otherwise it is paradoxical, contradictory and ridiculous, and shows the joints and seams where it has been fitted into the older account.

"But," you may ask, "what of the Messianic Prophecy mentioned by Matthew (1:23)? Surely this is a direct reference to the prophecy of Isaiah 7:14." Let us examine this so-called "prophecy," of which so much has been said and see just what reference it has to the birth of Jesus.

Turning back to Isaiah 7, we find these words, just a little before the "prophecy":

"Moreover the Lord spake again unto Ahaz, saying, Ask thee a sign of the Lord thy God; ask it either in the depth, or in the height above. But Ahaz said, I will not ask, neither will I tempt the Lord. And he said, Hear ye now, O house of David; is it a small thing for you to weary men, but will ye weary my God also?" (Isaiah 6:13.)

Then comes the "prophecy": "Therefore the Lord himself shall give you a sign; Behold a virgin shall conceive and bear a son and shall call his name Immanuel." This is the "prophecy" quoted by the writer of the Gospel of Matthew, and which has been quoted for centuries in Christian churches, as a foretelling of the miraculous birth of Jesus. As a matter of fact, intelligent theologians know that it has no reference to Jesus at all, in any way, but belongs to another occurrence, as we shall see presently, and was injected into the Gospel narrative merely to support the views of the writer thereof.

It may be well to add here that many of the best authorities hold that the Greek translation of the Hebrew word "almah" into the equivalent of "virgin" in the usual sense of the word is incorrect. The Hebrew word "almah" used in the original Hebrew text of Isaiah, does not mean "virgin" as the term is usually employed, but rather "a young woman of marriageable age—a maiden," the Hebrews having an entirely different word for the idea of "virginity," as the term is generally used. The word "almah" is used in other parts of the Old Testament to indicate a "young woman—a maiden," notably in Proverbs 30:19, in the reference to "the way of a man with a maid."

But we need not enter into discussions of this kind, say the Higher Critics, for the so-called "prophecy" refers to an entirely different matter. It appears, say they, that Ahaz, a weakling king of Judea, was in sore distress because Rezin the Syrian king, and Pekah the ruler of Northern Israel, had formed an offensive alliance against him and were moving their combined forces toward Jerusalem. In his fear he sought an alliance with Assyria, which alliance was disapproved of by Isaiah who remonstrated with Ahaz about the proposed move. The king was too much unnerved by fear to listen to Isaiah's arguments and so the latter dropped into prophecy. He prophesied, after the manner of the Oriental seer, that the land would be laid waste and misery entailed upon Israel, should the suicidal policy be adopted. But he held out a hope for a brighter future after the clouds of adversity had rolled by. A new and wise prince would arise who would bring Israel to her former glory. That prince would be born of a young mother and his name would be Immanuel, which means "God with us." All this had reference to things of a reasonably near future and had no reference to the birth of Jesus some seven hundred years after, who was not a prince sitting upon the throne of Israel, and who did not bring national glory and renown to Israel, for such was not his mission. Hebrew scholars and churchmen have often claimed that Isaiah's prophecy was fulfilled by the birth of Hezekiah.

There is no evidence whatever in the Jewish history of the seven hundred years between Isaiah and Jesus, that the Hebrews regarded Isaiah's prophecy as relating to the expected Messiah, but on the contrary it was thought to relate to a minor event in their history. As a Jewish writer has truly said, "Throughout the wide extent of Jewish literature there is not a single passage which can bear the construction that the Messiah should be miraculously conceived." Other writers along this line have stated the same thing, showing that the idea of a Virgin Birth was foreign to the Jewish mind, the Hebrews having always respected and highly honored married life and human parentage, regarding their children as blessings and gifts from God.

Another writer in the Church has said, "Such a fable as the birth of the Messiah from a virgin could have arisen anywhere else easier than among the Jews; their doctrine of the divine unity placed an impassable gulf between God and the world; their high regard for the marriage relation," etc., would have rendered the idea obnoxious. Other authorities agree with this idea, and insist that the idea of the Virgin Birth never originated in Hebrew prophecy, but was injected into the Christian Doctrine from pagan sources, toward the end of the first century, and received credence owing to the influx of converts from the "heathen" peoples who found in the idea a correspondence with their former beliefs. As Rev. R.J. Campbell, minister of the City Temple, London, says in his "New Theology," "No New Testament passage whatever is directly or indirectly a prophecy of the virgin birth of Jesus. To insist upon this may seem to many like beating a man of straw, but if so, the man of straw still retains a good deal of vitality."

Let us now turn to the second account of the Virgin Birth, in the Gospels—the only other place that it is mentioned, outside of the story in Matthew, above considered. We find this second mention in Luke 1:26-35, the verses having been quoted in the first part of this lesson.

There has been much dispute regarding the real authorship of the Gospel commonly accredited to Luke, but it is generally agreed upon by Biblical scholars that it was the latest of the first three Gospels (generally known as "the Synoptic Gospels"). It is also generally agreed upon, by such scholars, that the author, whoever he may have been, was not an eye witness of the events in the Life of Christ. Some of the best authorities hold that he was a Gentile (non-Hebrew), probably a Greek, for his Greek literary style is far above the average, his vocabulary being very rich and his diction admirable. It is also generally believed that the same hand wrote the Book of Acts. Tradition holds that the author was one Luke, a Christian convert after the death of Jesus, who was one of Paul's missionary band which traveled from Troas to Macedonia, and who shared Paul's imprisonment in Caesarea; and who shared Paul's shipwreck experiences on the voyage to Rome. He is thought to have written his Gospel long after the death of Paul, for the benefit and instruction of one Theophilus, a man of rank residing in Antioch.

It is held by writers of the Higher Criticism that the account of the Virgin Birth was either injected in Luke's narrative, by some later writer, or else that Luke in his old age adopted this view which was beginning to gain credence among the converted Christians of pagan origin, Luke himself being of this class. It is pointed out that as Paul, who was Luke's close friend and teacher, made no mention of the Virgin Birth, and taught nothing of the kind, Luke must have acquired the legend later, if, indeed, the narrative was written by him at all in his Gospel.

It is likewise noted that Luke also gives a genealogy of Jesus, from Adam, through Abraham, and David, and Joseph. The words in parenthesis "as was supposed," in Luke 3:23, are supposed to have been inserted in the text by a later writer, as there would be no sense or reason in tracing the genealogy of Jesus through a "supposed" father. The verse in question reads thusly: "And Jesus himself began to be about thirty years of age, being (as was supposed) the son of Joseph, which was the son of Heli," etc. Students, of course, notice that the line of descent given by Luke differs very materially from that given by Matthew, showing a lack of knowledge on the part of one or the other writer.

On the whole, scholars consider it most remarkable that this account of the Virgin Birth should be given by Luke, who was a most ardent Pauline student and follower, in view of the fact that Paul ignored the whole legend, if, indeed, he had ever heard of it. Surely a man like Paul would have laid great stress upon this wonderful event had he believed in it, or had it formed a part of the Christian Doctrine of his time. That Luke should have written this account is a great mystery—and many feel that it is much easier to accept the theory of the later interpolation of the story into Luke's Gospel, particularly in view of the corroborative indications.

Summing up the views of the Higher Criticism, we may say that the general position taken by the opponents and deniers of the Virgin Birth of Jesus is about as follows:

1. The story of the Virgin Birth is found only in the introductory portion of two of the four Gospels—Matthew and Luke—and even in these the story bears the appearance of having been "fitted in" by later writers.

2. Even Matthew and Luke are silent about the matter after the statements in the introductory part of their Gospels, which could scarcely occur had the story been written by and believed in by the writers, such action on their part being contrary to human custom and probability.

3. The Gospels of Mark and John are absolutely silent on the subject; the oldest of the Gospels—that of Mark—bears no trace of the legend; and the latest Gospel—that of John—being equally free from its mention.

4. The rest of the New Testament breathes not a word of the story or doctrine. The Book of Acts, generally accepted as having also been written by Luke, ignores the subject completely. Paul, the teacher of Luke, and the great writer of the Early Church, seems to know nothing

whatever about the Virgin Birth, or else purposely ignores it entirely, the latter being unbelievable in such a man. Peter, the First Apostle, makes no mention of the story or doctrine in his great Epistles, which fact is inconceivable if he knew of and believed in the legend. The Book of Revelation is likewise silent upon this doctrine which played so important a part in the later history of the Church. The great writings of the New Testament contain no mention of the story, outside of the brief mention in Matthew and Luke, alluded to above.

5. There are many verses in the Gospels and Epistles which go to prove, either that the story was unknown to the writers, or else not accepted by them. The genealogies of Joseph are cited to prove the descent of Jesus from David, which depends entirely upon the fact of Joseph's actual parentage. Jesus is repeatedly and freely mentioned as the son of Joseph. Paul and the other Apostles hold firmly to the doctrine of the necessity of the Death of Jesus; his Rising from the Dead; and his Ascension into Heaven, etc. But they had nothing to say regarding any necessity for his Virgin Birth, or the necessity for the acceptance of any such doctrine—they are absolutely silent on this point, although they were careful men, omitting no important detail of doctrine. Paul even speaks of Jesus as "of the seed of David." (Rom. 1:3.)

6. The Virgin Birth was not a part of the early traditions or doctrine of the Church, but was unknown to it. And it is not referred to in the preaching and teaching of the Apostles, as may have been seen by reference to the Book of Acts. This book, which relates the Acts and Teachings of the Apostles, could not have inadvertently omitted such an important doctrine or point of teaching. It is urged by careful and conscientious Christian scholars that the multitudes converted to Christianity in the early days must have been ignorant of, or uninformed on, this miraculous event, which would seem inexcusable on the part of the Apostles had they known of it and believed in its truth. This condition of affairs must have lasted until nearly the second century, when the pagan beliefs began to filter in by reason of the great influx of pagan converts.

7. There is every reason for believing that the legend arose from other pagan legends, the religions of other

peoples being filled with accounts of miraculous births of heroes, gods, and prophets, kings and sages.

8. That acceptance of the legend is not, nor should it be, a proof of belief in Christ and Christianity. This view is well voiced by Rev. Dr. Campbell, in his "New Theology," when he says "The credibility and significance of Christianity are in no way affected by the doctrine of the Virgin Birth, otherwise than that the belief tends to put a barrier between Jesus and the race, and to make him something that cannot properly be called human.... Like many others, I used to take the position that acceptance or non-acceptance of the doctrine of the Virgin Birth was immaterial because Christianity was quite independent of it; but later reflection has convinced me that in point of fact it operates as a hindrance to spiritual religion and a real living faith in Jesus. The simple and natural conclusion is that Jesus was the child of Joseph and Mary, and had an uneventful childhood." The German theologian, Soltau, says, "Whoever makes the further demand that an evangelical Christian shall believe in the words 'conceived by the Holy Ghost, born of the Virgin Mary,' wittingly constitutes himself a sharer in a sin against the Holy Spirit and the true Gospel as transmitted to us by the Apostles and their school in the Apostolic Age."

And this then is the summing up of the contention between the conservative school of Christian theologians on the one side and the liberal and radical schools on the other side. We have given you a statement of the positions, merely that you may understand the problem. But, before we pass to the consideration of the Occult Teachings, let us ask one question: How do the Higher Critics account for the undoubted doctrine of the Divine Fatherhood, as clearly stated all through the New Testament, in view of the proofs against the Virgin Birth? Why the frequent and repeated mention of Jesus as "the Son of God?" What was the Secret Doctrine underlying the Divine Parentage of Jesus, which the pagan legends corrupted into the story of the Virgin Birth of theology? We fear that the answer is not to be found in the books and preachments of the Higher Criticism, nor yet in those of the Conservative Theologians. Let us now see what light the Occult Teachings can throw on this dark subject! There is an Inner Doctrine which explains the mystery.

Now, in the first place, there is no reference in the Occult

Teaching to any miraculous features connected with the physical birth of Jesus. It is not expressly denied, it is true, but the Teachings contain no reference to the matter, and all the references to the subject of Jesus' parentage speak of Joseph as being His father, and Mary His mother. In other words, the family is treated as being composed of father, mother and child just as is the case with any family. The Occult Teachings go into great detail concerning the Spiritual Sonship of Jesus, as we shall see presently, but there is no mention of any miraculous physical conception and birth.

We can readily understand why the Virgin Birth legend would not appeal to the Occultists, if we will but consider the doctrines of the latter. The Occultists pay but little attention to the physical body, except as a Temple of the Spirit, and a habitation of the soul. The physical body, to the Occultist, is a mere material shell, constantly changing its constituent cells, serving to house the soul of the individual, and which when cast off and discarded is no more than any other bit of disintegrating material. They know of the existence of the soul separate from the body, both after the death of the latter and even during its life, in the case of Astral Travel, etc. And in many other ways it becomes natural for the Occultist to regard his body, and the bodies of others, as mere "shells," to be treated well, used properly, and then willingly discarded or exchanged for another.

In view of the above facts, you may readily see that any theory or doctrine which made the Absolute—God—overshadow a human woman's body and cause her to physically conceive a child, would appear crude, barbarous, unnecessary and in defiance of the natural laws established by the Cause of Causes. The Occultist sees in the conception of every child, the work of the Divine Will—every conception and birth a miracle. But he sees Natural Law underlying each, and he believes that the Divine Will always operates under Natural Laws—the seeming miracles and exceptions thereto, resulting from the mastery and operation of some law not generally known. But the Occultist knows of no law that will operate to produce conception by other than the physiological process.

In short, the Occultist does not regard the physical body of Jesus as Jesus Himself—he knows that the Real Jesus is something much greater than His body, and, consequently, he sees no more necessity for a miraculous conception of His body than he would for a miraculous creation of His robe. The body of Jesus was only material substance—the Real Jesus was Spirit. The Occultists do not regard Joseph as the father of the Real Jesus—no human being can produce or create a soul. And so, the Occultist sees no reason for accepting the old pagan doctrine of the physical Virgin Birth which has crept into Christianity from outside sources. To the Occultist, there is a real Virgin Birth of an entirely different nature, as we shall see presently.

But, not so with the people who flocked to the ranks of Christianity toward the close of the first century—coming from pagan people, and bringing with them their pagan legends and doctrines. These people believed that the Body was the Real Man, and consequently attached the greatest importance to it. These people were almost materialists as the result of their pagan views of life. They began to exert an influence on the small body of original Christians, and soon the original teachings were smothered by the weight of the pagan doctrines. For instance, they failed to grasp the beautiful ideas of Immortality held by the original Christians, which held that the soul survived the death and disintegration of the body. They could not grasp this transcendental truth—they did not know what was meant by the term "the soul," and so they substituted their pagan doctrine of the resurrection of the physical body. They believed that at some future time there would come a great Day, in which the Dead would arise from their graves, and become again alive. The crudeness of this idea, when compared to the beautiful doctrine of the Immortality of the Soul of the original Christians, and by the advanced Christians to-day, is quite painful. And yet these pagan converts actually smothered out the true teachings by their crude doctrine of resurrection of the body.

These people could not understand how a man could live without his physical body, and to them future life meant a resurrection of their dead bodies which would again become alive. To them the dead bodies would remain dead, until the Great Day, when they would be made alive again. There is no teaching among these people regarding the soul which passes out of the body and lives again on higher planes. No, nothing of this kind was known to these people—they were incapable of such high ideas and ideals—they were materialists and were wedded to their beloved animal bodies, and believed that their dead bodies would in some miraculous way be made alive again at some time in the future, when they would again live on earth.

In view of modern knowledge regarding the nature of matter, and the fact that what is one person's body to-day, may be a part of another's to-morrow—that matter is constantly being converted and reconverted—that the universal material is used to form bodies of animals, plants, men, or else dwell in chemical gases, or combinations in inorganic things—in view of these accepted truths the "resurrection of the body" seems a pitiful invention of the minds of a primitive and ignorant people, and not a high spiritual teaching. In fact, there may be many of you who would doubt that the Christians of that day so taught, were it not for the undisputed historical records, and the remnant of the doctrine itself embalmed in the "Apostle's Creed," in the passage "I believe in the resurrection of the body" which is read in the Churches daily, but which doctrine is scarcely ever taught in these days, and is believed in by but few Christians—in fact, is ignored or even denied by the majority.

Dr. James Beattie has written, "Though mankind have at all times had a persuasion of the immortality of the soul, the resurrection of the body was a doctrine peculiar to early Christianity." S.T. Coleridge has written, "Some of the most influential of the early Christian writers were materialists, holding the soul to be material—corporeal. It appears that in those days some few held the soul to be incorporeal, according to the views of Plato and others, but that the orthodox Christian divines looked upon this as an impious, unscriptural opinion. Justin Martyr argued against the Platonic nature of the soul. And even some latter-day writers have not hesitated to express their views on the subject, agreeing with the earlier orthodox brethren. For instance, Dr. R.S. Candlish has said,

> "You live again in the body,—in the very body, as to all essential properties, and to all practical intents and purposes, in which you live now. I am not to live as a ghost, a spectre, a spirit, I am to live then as I live now, in the body."

The reason that the early Church laid so much stress on this doctrine of the Resurrection of the Body, was because an inner sect, the Gnostics, held to the contrary, and the partisan spirit of the majority swung them to the other extreme, until they utterly denied any other idea, and insisted upon the resurrection and re-vitalizing of the physical body. But, in spite of the official fostering of this crude theory, it gradually sank into actual insignificance, although its shadow still persists in creed and word. Its spirit has retreated and passed away before the advancing idea of the Immortality of the Soul which returned again and again to Christianity until it won the victory. And as Prof. Nathaniel Schmidt has said, in his article on the subject in a leading encyclopaedia, "... The doctrine of the natural immortality of the human soul became so important a part of Christian thought that the resurrection naturally lost its vital significance, and it has practically held no place in the great systems of philosophy elaborated by the Christian thinkers in modern times." And, yet, the Church continues to repeat the now meaningless words, "I believe in the Resurrection of the Body." And while practically no one now believes it, still the recital of the words, and the statement of one's belief in them, forms a necessary requisite for admission into the Christian Church to-day. Such is the persistent hold of dead forms, and thoughts, upon living people.

And, so you can readily see from what has been said, why the early Christians, about the close of the first century A.D., attached so much importance to the physical conception and birth of Jesus. To them the physical body of Jesus was Jesus Himself. The rest follows naturally, including the Virgin Birth and the Physical Resurrection. We trust that you now understand this part of the subject.

We have heard devout Christians shocked at the idea that Jesus was born of a human father and mother, in the natural way of the race. They seemed to think that it savored of impurity. Such a notion is the result of a perverted idea of the sacredness of natural functions—a seeing of impurity—where all is pure. What a perversion, this regarding the sacredness of human Fatherhood, and Motherhood, as impure! The man of true spirituality sees in the Divine Trinity of Father, Mother and Child, something most pure and sacred—something that brings man very close indeed to God. Is the beautiful babe, held close in its mother's fond embrace, a symbol and type of impurity? Is the watchful care and love of the Father of the babe, an impure result of an impure cause? Does not one's own heart tell him the contrary? Look at the well known picture of the Journey to Egypt, with Mary carrying the babe, and both guarded and protected by the husband and father—Joseph—is this not a beautiful symbol of the sacredness of Parenthood? We trust that the majority of those who read these pages have advanced spiritually beyond the point where The Family is a thing of impure suggestion and relationship.

And, now, what are the Occult Teachings—the Secret Doctrine—regarding the Real Virgin Birth of Jesus? Just this: that the Spirit of Jesus was fresh from the bosom of the Absolute—Spirit of SPIRIT—a Virgin Birth of Spirit. His Spirit had not traveled the weary upward path of Reincarnation and repeated Rebirth, but was Virgin Spirit fresh from the SPIRIT—a very Son of the Father—

begotten not created. This Virgin Spirit was incarnated in His body, and there began the life of Man, not fully aware of His own nature, but gradually awakening into knowledge just as does every human soul, until at last the true nature of His Being burst upon him, and he saw that he indeed was God incarnate. In his short life of thirty-three years—thirty years of preparation, and three years of ministry, Jesus typified and symbolized the Life of the Race. Just as he awakened into a perception of his Divine Nature, so shall the race awaken in time. Every act in the Life of Jesus typified and symbolized the life of every individual soul, and of the race. We all have our Garden of Gethsemane—each is Crucified, and Ascends to Higher Planes. This is the Occult Doctrine of the Virgin Birth of Christ. Is it not a worthy one—is it not at least a higher conception of the human mind, than the physical Virgin Birth legend?

As we proceed with our lessons, we shall bring out the details of the Occult Teachings concerning the Divine Nature of Christ—the Spirit within the Human Form. And, in these references and instruction, you will see even more clearly that nature of the Spiritual Virgin Birth of Jesus.

The original Christians were instructed in the Truth concerning the Virgin Birth, that is, those who were sufficiently intelligent to grasp it. But after the great Teachers passed away, and their successors became overzealous in their desire to convert the outside peoples, the influx of the latter gradually overcame the original teachings, and the physical Virgin Birth and the Resurrection of the Body, became Doctrines and Articles of Faith, held of vital importance by the new orthodox leaders. It has taken centuries of mental struggle, and spiritual unfoldment to bring the Light of the Truth to bear upon this dark corner of the Faith, but the work is now fairly under way, and the great minds in the Church, as well as those out of the Church, are beginning to lay the old legend aside as a worn out relic of primitive days when the cloud of Ignorance overshadowed the Light of Truth.

In concluding this lesson, let us glance once more at the words of the eminent divine, Dr. Campbell, in his New Theology, in which he states:

> "But why hesitate about the question? The greatness of Jesus and the value of his revelation to mankind are in no way either assisted or diminished by the manner of his entry into the world. Every birth is just as wonderful as a virgin birth could possibly be, and just as much a direct act of God. A supernatural conception bears no relation

whatever to the moral and spiritual worth of the person who is supposed to enter the world in this abnormal way.... Those who insist on the doctrine will find themselves in danger of proving too much, for pressed to its logical conclusion, it removes Jesus altogether from the category of humanity in any real sense."

Let us trust that these Higher Critics may become informed upon the truths of the Occult Teachings, which supply the Missing Key, and afford the Reconciliation, and which show how and why Jesus is, in all and very truth, THE SON OF GOD, begotten and not created, of one substance from the Father—a particle of Purest Spirit fresh from the Ocean of Spirit, and free from the Karma of past Incarnations—how He was human and yet more than human.

In our next lesson we shall take up the narrative of the secret life of Jesus from the time of his appearance, as a child at the Temple, among the Elders, until when at the age of thirty years he appeared at the scene of the ministry of John the Baptist, and began his own brief ministry of three years which was closed by the Crucifixion and Ascension. This is a phase of the subject of intense interest, and startling nature, because of the lack of knowledge of the occult traditions on the part of the general public.

THE THIRD LESSON

THE MYSTIC YOUTH OF JESUS

In our last lesson we promised to tell you the esoteric story of the youth of Jesus. And there is such a story to tell, although the churches know little or nothing about it. The churches have nothing but the husks that have always been the property of the masses. The real kernels of truth have been possessed by but the few elect ones. The legends of the mystic brotherhoods and occult orders have preserved the story intact, and you shall now be given the essence of the mystic legends and traditions.

At the end of our first lesson we left Joseph, Mary and the infant Jesus in Egypt, the land to which they had flown to escape the wrath of the tyrant Herod. They dwelt in Egypt for a few years, until the death of Herod. Then Joseph retraced his steps, and returned toward his own country, bringing with him his wife and the babe. For some reasons unknown to those familiar with the legends and traditions, Joseph decided not to locate in Judea, but instead, bent his way toward the coast and returned to Nazareth where Mary and he had originally met and become betrothed. And, so, in Nazareth, the humble little mountain town the boyhood days of Jesus were spent, the grinding poverty of the family being relieved (according to the occult legends) by the yearly presents of gold from the hands of disguised messengers of the Magi.

The traditions relate that Jesus began His study of the Hebrew Law when He was but five years of age. It is related that He displayed an unusual ability and talent in the direction of mastering not only the text, but also the spirit of the Hebrew Scripture, and far outstripped His fellow students. It is also related that He displayed an early impatience at the dreary formalism of His Hebrew teachers, and a disposition to go right to the heart of the text before Him, that He might discern the spirit animating it. So much was this the case that He frequently brought down upon His head the censure of His instructors who overlooked the spirit of the teachings in their devotion to the forms and words.

Nazareth was an old-fashioned place and it and its inhabitants were made the target for the jests and witticisms of the people of Judea. The word "Nazarene" was synonymous with "lout"; "boor"; "peasant"; etc., to the residents of the more fashionable regions. The very remoteness of the town served to separate it in spirit from the rest of the country. But this very remoteness played an important part in the early life of Jesus. Nazareth, by reason of its peculiar location, was on the line of several caravan routes. Travelers from many lands traveled through the town, and rested there overnight, or sometimes for several days. Travelers from Samaria, Jerusalem, Damascus, Greece, Rome, Arabia, Syria, Persia, Phoenicia, and other lands mingled with the Nazarenes. And the traditions relate that Jesus, the child, would steal away and talk with such of these travelers as were versed in occult and mystic lore, and would imbibe from their varied founts of learning, until He was as thoroughly informed on these subjects as many a mystic of middle age. The traditions have it that the boy would often delight and astonish these traveling occultists with His wonderful insight into their secret doctrines and knowledge. And it is also told that some of the wisest of these, seeing the nature of the child, would overstay their allotted time of sojourn, that they might add here and there to the various parts of general occult lore possessed by the child. It is also taught that the Magi informed some of these travelers regarding the boy, that they might impart to him some truth or teaching for which He was ready.

And so the boy grew in knowledge and wisdom, day by day, year by year, until, finally, there occurred an event in His life, which has since been the subject of greatest interest to all Christians and students of the New Testament, but which without the above explanation is not readily understood.

The Feast of the Passover occurred in its allotted time of the year—April—when Jesus was in his thirteenth year. This feast was one of the most important in the Jewish calendar, and its observance was held as a most sacred duty by all Hebrews. It was the feast set down for the remembrance and perpetuation of that most important event in the history of the Jewish people when the Angel of Death swept over all of Egypt's land smiting the first-born child of every house of the natives, high and low, but sparing all the houses of the captive Hebrews who marked their door-sills with the sacrificial blood as a token of their faith. This is no place to give the explanation of this apparently miraculous event, which students now know to be due to natural causes. We merely mention it in passing.

The Law-givers of Israel had appointed the Feast of the Passover as a perpetual symbol of this event so important by the nation, and every self-respecting Jew felt obligated to take part in the observance and sacrament. Every pious Jew made it a point to perform a pilgrimage to Jerusalem at the time of the Feast of the Passover, if he could in any way manage to do so.

At the time of the Passover celebration of which we are speaking, Jesus had just entered into His thirteenth year, which age entitled Him, under the ecclesiastical law, to the privilege of sitting with the adult men of His race at the Passover supper, and also to publicly join with the male congregation in the thanksgiving service in the synagogues.

And so, on this year, He accompanied His father and mother to Jerusalem and made His second visit to the Holy City. It will be remembered that His first visit there was made when as an infant He was carried thither from Bethlehem in His mother's arms in accordance with the Jewish law, and at which time an aged priest and an old prophetess had publicly acknowledged the divine nature of the child.

The father, mother and child—the divine trinity of Human relationship—traveled slowly over the highway that led from Nazareth to Jerusalem. The father and mother were concerned with the details of the journey, mingled with pious thoughts concerning the sacred feast in which they were to take part. But the boy's mind was far away from the things that were occupying his parent's thoughts. He was thinking over the deep mystic truths which He had so readily absorbed during the past few years, and He was looking forward in delightful anticipation to His expected meeting with the older mystics in the temples and public places of Jerusalem.

It must be remembered that underlying the Jewish ecclesiastical teachings and formalism, which were all that the mass of the people knew, there was a great store of Jewish occultism and Mysticism known to the few elect. The Kaballah or Jewish occult writings were closely studied by the learned Jews, and this work with other similar teachings were transmitted verbally from teacher to student, and constituted the Secret Doctrine of the Hebrew religion. And it was toward the learned teachers of this Secret Doctrine that Jesus directed His mind and steps, although His parents knew it not.

Four or five days were consumed in the journey, and at last the Holy City—Jerusalem—came into full view, the wonderful Temple of Israel showing plainly above the other buildings. The bands of pilgrims, of which the family of Joseph formed a part, formed into orderly array and led by flute-players they solemnly marched into the streets of the Holy City, singing and chanting the Sacred Songs used by the faithful upon this solemn occasion. And the boy walked with the rest, with bowed head, and eyes that seemed to see things far removed from the scene around them.

The Passover rites were carried out—the duties were performed—the ceremonies were observed. The Passover Feast extended over a full week, of which the first two days were the most important, and during which two days the obligatory ceremonies were performed. Each family made the offering of the sacrificial lamb—each family baked and ate the unleavened bread. The beautiful idea of the Passover had degenerated into a horrible feast of blood, for it is related that upon these occasions over a quarter-million of poor innocent lambs were slaughtered and offered up as a sacrifice pleasing to Jehovah, who was supposed to delight in this flood of the blood of innocents. In pursuance of this barbarous idea, the altars and courts of the Temple of the Living God ran red with the life-blood of these poor creatures, and the hands and garments of the anointed priests of Jehovah were stained like those of butchers, that the vanity of a barbarous conception of Deity might be fed.

All this for "the Glory of God!" Think of it! And think of the feeling that must have been aroused in the mystic mind of Jesus at this horrible sight. How His soul must have been outraged at this prostitution of the sacred rite! And what would have been His thoughts had He known that centuries after, a great religion would stand, bearing His name, the followers of which would be carried away with this same false idea of sacrificial blood, which would be voiced in hymns about "A fountain filled with blood, flowing from Immanuel's veins," and about "sinners plunged beneath that bloody flood losing all their guilty stains?" Alas, for the prostitution of sacred truths and teachings. No wonder that a people so saturated with the abominable ideas of a Deity delighting in this flow of blood should have afterward put to death the greatest man of their race—a Being who came to bring them the highest mystic and occult truths. And their prototypes have survived through the centuries, even unto today, insisting upon this idea of blood sacrifice and death atonement, unworthy of any people except the worshipers of some heathen devil-god in the remote sections of darkest Africa.

Disgusted and outraged by this barbarous sight, Jesus, the boy, stole away from the side of His parents, and sought the remote chambers and corridors of the Temple where were to be found the great teachers of the Law and of the Kaballah, surrounded by their students. Here the boy sat and listened to the teachings and disputations of the teachers and exponents of the doctrines. From one group to another He wandered, and listened, and pondered, and thought. He compared the teachings, and submitted the various ideas to the touchstone of the truth as He found it within His own mind. The hours rapidly passed by unnoticed by the boy, who found Himself amidst such congenial environments for the first time. The talks with the travelers of the caravans paled into insignificance when compared with these of the great occult teachers of Israel. For be it remembered that it was the custom of the great teachers of that day to so instruct those who were attracted to their company. And Jerusalem being the centre of the culture and learning of Israel, the great teachers dwelt there. And so it will be seen that Jesus now found Himself at the very fountain-head of the Hebrew Secret Doctrines, and in the actual presence of the great teachers.

On the third day, there began a breaking-up of the vast gathering of the two million of people who had made the pilgrimage to the Holy City. Those poorer in purse were the first to leave, after the obligatory rites of the first two days had been performed. And Joseph and Mary were among those preparing to retrace their steps to their distant homes. Their friends and neighbors gathered together, and the preparations for the return were completed. But at the last moment, the parents discovered that the boy, Jesus, was missing. They were alarmed, but friends told them that their boy had been seen in the company of kinsmen and neighbors traveling along the same road, who had preceded them but a few hours. Somewhat reassured, the parents left with their company, hoping that they would overtake the boy before nightfall. But when they reached the first station on the caravan route—a village called Beroth—and the night descended upon them, and the boy failed to appear among the neighbors and kinsmen, the parents were sorely distressed. They slept but little that night, and when the first rays of dawn appeared, they parted from the company, and retraced their way back to Jerusalem, in search of the boy apparently lost in the great capital amid the hundreds of thousands of pilgrims.

Every mother and father will enter into the feelings of Joseph and Mary in their frantic return to the city, and in their subsequent search for the lost child. They inquired here and there for the boy, but not a trace of him was found. And night came without a ray of hope. And the next day was likewise barren of results. And the next day after. For three days the devoted parents searched high and low for their beloved child—but no word of encouragement came to them. The boy had seemingly dropped out of sight in the vast crowds and winding streets. The parents reproached themselves for their lack of care and caution. None but a parent can imagine their anguish and terror.

They visited the many courts of the Temple many times, but no sight or word of the boy rewarded their search. The bloody altars, the showy costumes of the priests; the chants; the readings; seemed like mockery to them. They wished themselves back in their humble village, with their boy by their side. They prayed and besought Jehovah to grant their hopes and desire, but no answer came.

Then, on the last day, a strange event occurred. The weary and heart broken parents wandered once more into the Temple—this time visiting one of the less frequented courts. They saw a crowd gathered—something of importance was occurring. Almost instinctively they drew near to the crowd. And then amidst the unusual silence of the people they heard a boyish voice raised to a pitch adapted to a large circle of hearers, and speaking in the tones of authority. It was the voice of the boy, Jesus!

With eager feet the couple pushed forward, unto the very inner row of the circle. And there, wonder of wonders, they saw their child in the centre of the most celebrated teachers and doctors of the Law in all Israel. With a rapt expression in his eyes, as if He were gazing upon things not of this world, the boy Jesus was standing in a position and attitude of authority, and around him were grouped the greatest minds of the day and land, in respectful attention, while at a further distance stood the great circle of the common people.

When one remembers the Jewish racial trait of reverence for age, and the consequent submission of Youth, one will better understand the unusual spectacle that burst upon the gaze of Joseph and Mary. A mere boy—a child—daring to even speak boldly in the presence of the aged teachers was unheard of, and the thought of such a one actually presuming to dispute, argue and teach, in such an assembly, was like unto a miracle. And such it was!

The boy spoke with the air and in the tones of a Master. He met the most subtle arguments and objections of the Elders with the power of the keenest intellect and spiritual insight. He brushed aside the sophistries with a contemptuous phrase, and brought back the argument to the vital point.

The crowd gathered in greater volume, the gray heads and beards grew more and more respectful. It was evident to all that a Master had arisen in Israel in the form of a boy of thirteen. The MASTER was apparent in tone, gesture, and thought. The Mystic had found his first audience, and his congregation was composed of the leading thinkers and teachers of the land. The insight of the Magi was verified!

Then in a momentary pause in the argument, the stifled cry of a woman was heard—the voice of the Mother. The crowd turned impatient, reproachful glances upon Mary, who had been unable to restrain her emotion. But the boy, looking sadly but affectionately at his lost parents, gave her a reassuring glance, which at the same time bade her remain still until he had finished his discourse. And the parents obeyed the newly awakened will of their child.

The teaching ended, the boy stepped from his position with the air of one of the Elders, and rejoined his parents, who passed as rapidly as possible from the wondering crowd. Then his mother reproached him, telling him of their distress and wearisome search. The boy listened calmly and patiently until she had finished. Then he asked, with his newly acquired air of authority, "Why sought ye me?" And when they answered him in the customary manner of parents, the boy took on still a greater air of authority, and in tones that though kindly, were full of power, he replied, "Knew ye not, that I must be in my Father's House? I must be about the things of my Father." And the parents, feeling themselves in the presence of the Mystery that had ever been about the child, followed Him silently from the Temple grounds.

And here closes the New Testament story of the boy Jesus at the age of thirteen, which story is not resumed until His appearance at the place of the preaching of John the Baptist, over seventeen years later, when the boy had reached the age of a man of thirty years. When and how did he spend those seventeen years? The New Testament is totally silent on this score. Can anyone who has read the above imagine that Jesus spent these years as a growing youth and young man, working at His father's carpenter bench in the village of Nazareth? Would not the Master, having found his strength and power, have insisted upon developing the same? Could the Divine Genius once self-recognized be content to be obscured amid material pursuits? The New Testament is silent, but the Occult Traditions and Mystic Legends tell us the story of the missing seventeen years, and these we shall now give to you.

* * * * *

The legends and traditions of the mystic and occult organizations and brotherhoods tell us that after the occurrence of Jesus and the Elders in the Temple, and his recovery by his parents, the latter were approached by members of the secret organization to which the Magi belonged, who pointed out to the parents the injustice of the plan of keeping the lad at the carpenter's bench when He had shown evidences of such a marvelous spiritual development and such a wonderful intellectual grasp of weighty subjects. It is told that after a long and serious consideration of the matter the parents finally consented to the plan advanced by the Magi, and allowed them to take the lad with them into their own land and retreats that He might there receive the instructions for which His soul craved, and for which His mind was fitted.

It is true that the New Testament does not corroborate these occult legends, but it is likewise true that it says nothing to the contrary. It is silent regarding this important period of between seventeen and eighteen years. It is to be remembered that when He appeared upon the scene of John's ministration, the latter did not recognize Him, whereas had Jesus remained about His home, John, his cousin, would have been acquainted with his features and personal appearance.

The occult teachings inform us that the seventeen or eighteen years of Jesus' life regarding which the Gospels are silent, were filled with travels in far and distant lands, where the youth and young man was instructed in the occult lore and wisdom of the different schools. It is taught that He was taken into India, and Egypt, and Persia, and other far regions, living for several years at each important center, and being initiated into the various brotherhoods, orders, and bodies having their headquarters there. Some of the Egyptians' orders have traditions of a young Master who sojourned among them, and such is likewise the case in Persia and in India. Even among the lamasaries hidden in Thibet and in the Himalayan Mountains are to be found legends and stories regarding the marvelous young Master who once visited there and absorbed their wisdom and secret knowledge.

More than this, there are traditions among the Brahmans, Buddhists and Zoroastrians, telling of a strange young teacher who appeared among them, who taught marvelous truths and who aroused great opposition among the priests of the various religions of India and Persia, owing to his preaching against priestcraft and formalism, and also by his bitter opposition to all forms of caste distinctions and restrictions. And this, too, is in accord with the occult legends which teach that from about the age of twenty-one until the age of nearly thirty years Jesus pursued a ministry among the people of India and Persia and neighboring countries, returning at last to his native land where He conducted a ministry extending over the last three years of His life.

The occult legends inform us that He aroused great interest among the people of each land visited by Him, and that He also aroused the most bitter opposition among the priests, for He always opposed formalism and priestcraft, and sought to lead the people back to the Spirit of the Truth, and away from the ceremonies and forms which have always served to dim and becloud the Light of the Spirit. He taught always the Fatherhood of God and the Brotherhood of Man. He sought to bring the great Occult Truths down to the comprehension of the masses of people who had lost the Spirit of the Truth in their observance of outward forms and pretentious ceremonies.

It is related that in India He brought down upon His head the wrath of the Brahmin upholders of the caste distinctions, that curse of India. He dwelt in the huts of the Sudras, the lowest of all of the Hindu castes, and was therefore regarded as a pariah by the higher classes. Everywhere He was regarded as a firebrand and a disturber of established social order by the priests and high-caste people. He was an agitator, a rebel, a religious renegade, a socialist, a dangerous man, an "undesirable citizen," to those in authority in those lands.

But the seeds of His wisdom were sown right and left, and in the Hindu religions of today, and in the teachings of other Oriental countries, may be found traces of Truth, the resemblance of which to the recorded teachings of Jesus, show that they came from the same source, and have sorely disturbed the Christian missionaries that have since visited these lands.

And so, slowly and patiently, Jesus wended his way homeward toward Israel, where He was to complete His ministry by three years' work among His own race, and where He was to again raise up against Himself the opposition of the priests and the upper classes which would finally result in His death. He was a rebel against the established order of things, and He met the fate reserved for those who live ahead of their time.

And, as from the first days of His ministry to His last, so it is today, the real teachings of the Man of Sorrows reach more readily the heart of the plain people, while they are reviled and combatted by those in ecclesiastical and temporal authority, even though these people claim allegiance to Him and wear His livery. He was ever the friend of the poor and oppressed, and hated by those in authority.

And so, you see the Occult teachings show Jesus to have been a world-wide teacher, instead of a mere Jewish prophet. The world was his audience, and all races His hearers.

He planted His seeds of Truth in the bosom of many religions instead of but one, and these seeds are beginning to bear their best fruit even now at this late day, when the truth of the Fatherhood of

God and the Brotherhood of Man is beginning to be felt by all nations alike, and is growing strong enough to break down the old which have divided brother from brother, and creed from creed. Christianity—true Christianity—is not a mere creed, but a great human and divine Truth that will rise above all petty distinctions of race and creed and will at last shine on all men alike, gathering them into one fold of Universal Brotherhood.

May the Great Day be hastened!

* * * * *

And so we leave Jesus, wending his way slowly homeward toward Judea, the land of His father and the place of His birth. Dropping a word here—planting a seed there—onward He pursued His way. Visiting this mystic brotherhood, and resting a while in another occult retreat, He slowly retraced the journey of His youth. But while His outward journey was that of a student traveling forth to complete His education, He returned as a Master and Teacher, bearing and sowing the seeds of a great Truth, which was to grow and bring forth great fruit, and which, in time, would spread over all the world in its primitive purity, notwithstanding its betrayal and corruption at the hands of those in whose keeping He left it when he passed away from the scene of His labors.

Jesus came as a World Prophet, not as a mere Jewish holyman, and still less as a Hebrew Messiah destined to sit upon the throne of His father David. And He left His mark upon all of the great peoples of earth by His journey among them. Throughout Persia are found many traditions of Issa, the young Master who appeared in that land centuries ago, and who taught the Fatherhood of God and the Brotherhood of Man. Among the Hindus are found strange traditions of Jesoph or Josa, a young ascetic, who passed through the Hind long since, denouncing the established laws of caste, and consorting with the common people, who, as in Israel, "heard him gladly." Even in China are found similar tales of the young religious firebrand, preaching ever the Brotherhood of Man—ever known as the Friend of the Poor. On and on He went, sowing the seeds of human freedom and the casting off of the yoke of ecclesiastical tyranny and formalism, which seeds are springing unto growth even at this late day. Yea, the Spirit of His real teachings are even now bearing fruit in the hearts of men, and though nearly two thousand years have passed by the "soul" of His social teachings still "goes marching on" round and round the world.

THE FOURTH LESSON

THE BEGINNING OF THE MINISTRY

When Jesus reached his native land, after the years of travel in India, Persia and Egypt, he is believed by the occultists to have spent at least one year among the various lodges and retreats of the Essenes. By reference to the first lesson of this series you will see who and what was this great mystic organization—the Essenic Brotherhood. While resting and studying in their retreats His attention was diverted to the work of Johannen—John the Baptist—and He saw there an opening wedge for the great work that He felt called upon to do among His own people. Dreams of converting His own race—the Jews—to His conception of Truth and Life, crept over Him, and he determined to make this work His great life task.

The feeling of race is hard to overcome and eradicate, and Jesus felt that, after all, here He was at last, at home, among His own people, and the ties of blood and race reasserted themselves. He put aside His previous thoughts of a world-wandering life, and decided to plant the standard of the Truth in Israel, so that from the capital of the Chosen People the Light of the Spirit might shine forth to all the world. It was Jesus the man—Jesus the Jew—that made this choice. From the broader, higher point of view He had no race; no country; no people;—but His man nature was too strong, and in yielding to it he sowed the seeds for His final undoing.

Had he merely passed through Judea as a traveling missionary, as had done many others before Him, he would have escaped the punishment of the government. Although He would have aroused the hatred and opposition of the priests, He would have not laid Himself open to the charge of wishing to become the King of the Jews, or the Jewish Messiah, come to resume the throne of David, His forefather. But it avails us nought to indulge in speculations of this kind, for who knows what part Destiny or Fate plays in the Great Universal plan—who knows where Free-Will terminates and Destiny moves the pieces on the board, that the Great Game of Universal Life be played according to the plan?

While among the Essenes, as we have said, Jesus first heard of John, and determined to use the ministry of the latter as an opening wedge for His own great work. He communicated to the Essenic Fathers His determination to travel to John's field of work later on, and the Fathers sent word of this to John. The legends have it that John did not know who was coming, being merely informed that a great Master from foreign parts would join him later on, and that he, John, should prepare the people for his coming.

And John followed these instructions from his superiors in the Essenic Brotherhood to the letter, as you will see by reference to our first lesson, and to the New Testament. He preached repentance; righteousness; the Essenic rite of Baptism; and above all the Coming of the Master. He bade his hearers repent—"repent ye! for the Kingdom of Heaven is at hand"!—"repent ye! for the Master cometh!" cried he in forceful tones.

And when his people gathered around him and asked whether he, John, were not indeed the Master, he answered them, saying, "Nay, I am not He whom thou seekest. After me there cometh one whose sandals I am not worthy to unloose. I baptize thee with water, but He shall baptize thee with the Fire of the Spirit that is within Him!" It was ever and always this exhortation toward fitness for the coming of the Master. John was a true Mystic, who sank his personality in the Work he was called on to do, and who was proud to be but the Forerunner of the Master, of whose coming he had been informed by the Brotherhood.

And, as we have told you in the first lesson, one day there came before him, a young man, of a dignified, calm appearance, gazing upon him with the expressive eyes of the true Mystic. The stranger asked to be baptized, but John, having perceived the occult rank of the stranger by means of the signs and symbols of the Brotherhood, rebelled at the Master receiving baptism at the hands of himself, one far below the occult rank of the stranger. But Jesus, the stranger, said to John, "Suffer it to be," and stepped into the water to receive the mystic rite again, as a token to the people that He had come as one of them.

And then occurred that strange event, with which you are familiar, when a dove descended as if from Heaven and rested over the head of the stranger, and a soft voice, even as the sighing of the wind through the trees, was heard, whispering, "This is my beloved son, in whom I am well pleased." And then the stranger, evidently awed by the strange message from the Beyond, passed away from the multitude, and bent his way toward the wilderness, as if in need of a retreat in which he could meditate over the events of the day, and regarding the work which He could now dimly see stretching its way before Him.

The average student of the New Testament passes over the event of Jesus in the Wilderness, with little or no emotion, regarding it as a mere incident in His early career. Not so with the mystic or occultist, who knows, from the teachings of his order, that in the Wilderness Jesus was subjected to a severe occult test, designed to develop His power, and test His endurance. In fact, as every advanced member of any of the great occult orders knows, the occult degree known as "The Ordeal of the Wilderness" is based upon this mystic experience of Jesus, and is intended to symbolize the tests to which He was subjected. Let us consider this event so fraught with meaning and importance to all true occultists.

The Wilderness toward which Jesus diverted His steps, lay afar off from the river in which the rites of Baptism had been performed. Leaving behind him the fertile banks, and acres, of cultivated land, He approached the terrible Wilderness which even the natives of that part of the country regarded with superstitious horror. It was one of the weirdest and dreariest spots in even that weird and dreary portion of the country. The Jews called it "The Abode of Horror"; "The Desolate Place of Terror"; "The Appalling Region"; and other names suggestive of the superstitious dread which it inspired in their hearts. The Mystery of the Desert Places hung heavy over this place, and none but the stoutest hearts ventured within its precincts. Though akin to the desert, the place abounded in dreary and forbidding hills, crags, ridges and canyons. Those of our readers who have ever traveled across the American continent and have seen some of the desolate places of the American Desert, and who have read of the terrors of Death Valley, or the Alkali Lands, may form an idea of the nature of this Wilderness toward which the Master was traveling.

All normal vegetation gradually disappeared as He pressed further and further into this terrible place, until naught remained but the scraggy vegetation peculiar to these waste places—those forms of plant life that in their struggle for existence had managed to survive under such adverse conditions as to give the naturalist the impression that the very laws of natural plant life have been defied and overcome.

Little by little the teeming animal life of the lower lands disappeared, until at last no signs of such life remained, other than the soaring vultures overhead and the occasional serpent and crawling things under foot. The silence of the waste places was upon the traveler, brooding heavily over Him and all around the places upon which He set His foot, descending more heavily upon Him each moment of His advance.

Then came a momentary break in the frightful scene. He passed through the last inhabited spot in the approach to the heart of the Wilderness—the tiny village of Engedi, where were located the ancient limestone reservoirs of water which supplied the lower regions of the territory. The few inhabitants of this remote outpost of primitive civilization gazed in wonder and awe at the lonely figure passing them with unseeing eyes and with gaze seemingly able to pierce the forbidding hills which loomed up in the distance hiding lonely recesses into which the foot of man had never trodden, even the boldest of the desert people being deterred from a visit thereto by the weird tales of unholy creatures and unhallowed things, which made these places the scene of their uncanny meetings and diabolical orgies.

On, and on, pressed the Master, giving but slight heed to the desolate scene which now showed naught but gloomy hills, dark canyons, and bare rocks, relieved only by the occasional bunches of stringy desert grass and weird forms of cacti bristling with the protective spines which is their armor against their enemies.

At last the wanderer reached the summit of one of the higher foot-hills and gazed at the scene spreading itself before Him. And that scene was one that would have affrighted the heart of an ordinary man. Behind Him was the country through which He had passed, which though black and discouraging was as a paradise to the country which lay ahead of Him. There below and behind Him were the caves and rude dwellings of the outlaws and fugitives from justice who had sought the doubtful advantage of security from the laws of man. And far away in the distance were the scenes of John the Baptist's ministry, where He could see in imagination the multitude discussing the advent of the strange Master, who had been vouched for by the Voice, but who had stolen swiftly away from the scene, and had fled the crowds who would have gladly worshipped Him as a Master and have obeyed His slightest command.

Then as the darkness of the succeeding nights fell upon Him, He would sleep on some wild mountain cliff, on the edge of some mighty precipice, the sides of which dropped down a thousand feet or more. But these things disturbed Him not. On and on He pressed at the appearance of each dawn. Without food He boldly moved forward to the Heart of the Hills, where the Spirit guided Him to the scene of some great spiritual struggle which he intuitively knew lay before Him.

The Words of the Voice haunted Him still, though He lacked a full understanding of them, for He had not yet unfolded the utmost recesses of His Spiritual Mind. "This is my Beloved Son, in whom I am well pleased"—what meant these words? And still, no answer came to that cry of His soul which sought in vain for a freeing of that riddle.

And still on and on He pressed, until at last He mounted the steep sides of the barren forbidding mountain of Quarantana, beyond which He felt that His struggle was to begin. No food was to be found—He must fight the battle unaided by the material sustenance that ordinary men find necessary for life and strength. And still He had not received the answer to the cry of His soul. The rocks beneath His feet—the blue sky above His head—the lofty peaks of Moab and Gilead in the distance—gave no answer to the fierce insistent desire for the answer to the Riddle of the Voice. The answer must come from Within, and from Himself only. And in the Heart of the Wilderness He must remain, without food, without shelter, without human companionship, until the Answer came. And as it was with the Master, so is it with the follower—all who attain the point of unfoldment at which the Answer is alone possible, must experience that awful feeling of "aloneness" and spiritual hunger, and frightful remoteness from all that the world values, before the Answer comes from Within—from the Holy of Holies of the Spirit.

* * * * *

To realize the nature of the spiritual struggle that awaited Jesus in the Wilderness—that struggle that would bring Him face to face with His own soul, we must understand the Jewish longing and expectation of the Messiah. The Messianic traditions had taken a strong hold upon the minds of the Jewish people, and it needed but the spark of a strong personality to set all Israel into a blaze which would burn fiercely and destroy the foreign influences which have smothered the national spirit. The idea of a Messiah springing from the loins of David, and coming to take His rightful place as the King of the Jews, was imbedded in the heart of every Jew worthy of the name. Israel was oppressed by its conquerors, and made subject to a foreign yoke, but when the Messiah would come to deliver Israel, every Jew would arise to drive out the foreign invaders and conquerors—the yoke of Rome would be thrown off, and Israel would once more take its place among the nations of the earth.

Jesus knew full well the fact of this national hope. It had been installed into His mind from childhood. He had pondered over it often during the time of His wanderings and sojourn in foreign lands. The occult legends, however, make no mention of His having ever thought of Himself as the Messiah until he was about to re-enter His own land after His years of foreign study and ministry. It is thought that the idea of His being the long expected Messiah was first suggested by some of the Essenic teachers, when He rested with them for awhile before appearing before John the Baptist. It was pointed out to Him that the marvelous events surrounding His birth indicated that He was a marked individual destined to play an important part in the history of the World. Then why was it not reasonable to believe that that role was to be that of the Messiah come to sit on the throne of His father David, and destined to bring Israel from her now obscure position to once more shine as a bright star in the firmament of nations? Why was it not reasonable that He was to lead the Chosen People to their own?

Jesus began to ponder over these things. He had absolutely no material ambitions for Himself and all His impulses and inclinations were for the life of an occult ascetic. But the idea of a redeemed and regenerated Israel was one calculated to fire the blood of any Jew, even though the element of personal ambition might be lacking in him.

He had always realized that in some way He was different from other men, and that some great work lay ahead of Him, but He had never understood His own nature, nor the work He was to do. And it is not to be wondered that the talk among the Essenes caused Him to ponder carefully over the idea expressed by them. And then the wonderful event of the dove, and the Voice, upon the occasion of His baptism, seemed almost to verify the idea of the Essenes. Was He indeed the long-expected Deliverer of Israel? Surely He must find this out—He must wring the answer from the inmost recesses of His soul. And so, He sought refuge in the Wilderness, intuitively feeling that there amidst the solitude and desolation, He would fight His fight and receive His answer.

He felt that He had come to a most important phase of His life's work, and the question of "What Am I?" must be settled, once and for all,—then and there. And so He left behind Him the admiring and worshipful crowds of John's following, and sought the solitude of the waste places of the Wilderness, in which He felt He would come face to face with His own soul, and demand and receive its answer.

* * * * *

And up in the inmost recesses of the Heart of the Wilderness, Jesus wrestled in spirit with Himself for many days, without food or nourishment, and without shelter. And the struggle was terrific—worthy of such a great soul. First the body's insistent needs were to be fought and mastered. It is related that the climax of the physical struggle came one day when the Instinctive Mind, which attends to the physical functions, made a desperate and final demand upon Him. It cried aloud for bread with all the force of its nature. It tempted Him with the fact that by His own occult powers He was able to convert the very stones into bread, and it demanded that He work the miracle for His own physical needs—a practice deemed most unworthy by all true occultists and mystics. "Turn this stone into bread, and eat" cried the voice of the Tempter. But Jesus resisted the temptation although He knew that by the power of His concentrated thought He had but first to mentally picture the stone as bread and then will that it be so materialized. The miraculous power which afterward turned water into wine, and which was again used to feed the multitude with the loaves and the fishes, was available to Him at that moment in order to satisfy the cravings of His body, and to break His fast.

None but the advanced occultist who has known what it was to be tempted to use his mysterious powers to satisfy his personal wants, can appreciate the nature of the struggle through which Jesus passed, and from which He emerged victorious. And like the occult Master that He was, He summoned His Inner Forces and beat off the Tempter.

* * * * *

But a still greater temptation than this arose to try Him to the utmost. He found Himself brought face to face with the idea of Messiahship, and Kingship of the Jews, of which we spoke. Was He the Messiah? And if so, what must be His course of life and action? Was He destined to throw aside the robe and staff of the ascetic, and to don the royal purple and the sceptre? Was He to forsake the role of the spiritual guide and teacher, and to become the King and Ruler over the people of Israel? These were the questions He asked His soul, and for which He demanded an answer.

And the mystic legends tell us that His Spirit answered by showing Him two sets of mental pictures, with the assurance that He could choose either, at will, and cause it to become realized.

The first picture showed Him true to His spiritual instincts, and loyal to His mission, but which rendered Him indeed the "Man of Sorrows." He saw himself continuing to sow the seeds of Truth, which would, centuries after, spring up, blossom and bear fruit to nourish the world, but which would now bring down upon His head the hatred and persecution of those in power and authority. And He saw each successive step, each showing the approach of the end, until at last He saw Himself crowned with thorns and meeting the death of a criminal on the cross, between two base criminals of the lowest classes of men. All this He saw and even His brave heart felt a deadly sickness at the ignominious end of it all—the apparent failure of His earthly mission. But it is related that some of the mighty intelligences which dwell upon the higher planes of existence, gathered around Him, and gave Him words of encouragement and hope and resolve. He found Himself literally in the midst of the Heavenly Host, and receiving the inspiration of its presence.

Then this picture—and the Host of Invisible Helpers—faded away, and the second picture began to appear before the vision of the lonely dweller of the Wilderness. He saw the picture of Himself descending the mountain, and announcing Himself as the Messiah—the King of the Jews—who had come to lead His Chosen People to victory and deliverance. He saw Himself acclaimed as the Promised One of Israel, and the multitude flocking to His banners. He saw Himself at the head of a great conquering army, marching toward Jerusalem. He saw Himself making use of His highly developed occult powers to read the minds of the enemy and thus know their every movement and intention, and the means to overcome them. He saw Himself miraculously arming and feeding His hosts of battle. He saw Himself smiting the enemy with His occult powers and forces. He saw the yoke of Rome being cast off, and its phalanxes fleeing across the borders in terror and disgraceful defeat. He saw Himself mounting the throne of David, His forefather. He saw Himself instituting a reign of the highest type, which would make of Israel the leading nation of the world. He saw Israel's sphere of influence extending in all directions, until Persia, Egypt, Greece and even the once-feared Rome, become tributary nations. He saw Himself in the triumphant chariot on some great feast day of victory, with Caesar himself tied to the tail of His chariot—a slave to Israel's King. He saw His royal court outrivaling that of Solomon, and becoming the center of the world. He saw Jerusalem as the capital of the world, and He, Jesus of Nazareth, son of David the King, as its Ruler, its hero, its demi-god. The very apotheosis of human success showed in the picture of Himself and His Beloved Israel in the picture.

And then the Temple was seen to be the Center of the Religious thought of the World. The Religion of the Jews, as modified by His own advanced views, would be the religion of all men. And he would be the favored mouthpiece of the God of Israel. All the dreams of the Hebrew Fathers would be realized in Him, the

Messiah of the New Israel whose capital would be Jerusalem, the Queen of the World.

And all this by simply the exercise of his occult powers under the direction of HIS WILL. It is related that accompanying this second picture and attracted by its mighty power, came all the great thought-waves of the world which had been thought by men of all times who thought and acted out the Dreams of Power. These clouds settled down upon Him like a heavy fog, and their vibrations were almost overpowering. And also came the hosts of the disembodied souls of those who while living had sought or gained power. And each strove to beat into His brain the Desire of Power. Never in the history of man have the Powers of Darkness so gathered together for attack upon the mind of a mortal man. Would it have been any wonder had even such a man as Jesus succumbed?

But He did not succumb. Rallying His Inner Force to His rescue He beat back the attacking horde, and by an effort of His Will, He swept both picture and tempters away into oblivion, crying indignantly "Thou darest to tempt even me, thy Lord and Master. Get thee behind me thou Fiends of Darkness"!

And so the Temptation of the Wilderness failed, and Jesus received His answer from His soul, and He descended the mountains, back to the haunts of men—back to the scene of His three years' labors and suffering, and back to His Death. And He knew full well all that awaited Him there, for had He not seen the First Picture?

Jesus had chosen His career.

* * * * *

The Master descended from the mountains and forsook the Wilderness for the place in which John and his followers were gathered. Resting for a time, and refreshing Himself with food and drink, He gathered together His energies for His great work.

The followers of John gathered around Him, filled with the idea that He was the Messiah come to lead them to victory and triumph. But He disappointed them by His calm, simple manner, and His disavowal of royal claims. "What seek ye of me?" he asked them, and many, abashed, left His circle and returned to the crowd. But a few humble souls remained and around these few gathered a few more, until at last a little band of faithful students was formed—the first band of Christian disciples. This band was composed almost entirely of fishermen and men of similar humble occupations. There was an absence of people of rank or social position. His people were of the "plain people" which have furnished the recruits for every great religion.

And after a time, Jesus moved away from the place, followed by His band of disciples, which drew new members from each place of gathering. Some stayed but for a short time, while others replaced the faint hearted ones of little faith. But the band steadily grew, until it began to attract the attention of the authorities and the public. Jesus constantly disclaimed being the Messiah, but the report that such indeed He was, began to spread and the authorities began that system of spying and watching which followed His footsteps for three years, and which finally resulted in His death on the Cross. And this suspicion was encouraged by the Jewish priesthood which began to hate the young teacher whose opposition to their tyranny and formalism was quite marked.

The band one day came to a small village in Galilee, and Jesus began His usual meetings and teaching. Near where they gathered was a house at which preparations were being made for a wedding feast. The wedding ceremony has always been an important occasion among the Jews. The most elaborate preparations consistent with the size of the purse of the girl's parents are indulged in. Relatives from far and near gather to the feast. Jesus happened to be a distant kinsman of the bride, and according to custom He was bidden to the feast.

The guests began to gather, each depositing his sandals in the outer court, and entering the guest chamber barefooted, after carefully bathing his feet and ankles after the custom still prevailing in Oriental countries. Jesus was accompanied by a few of His faithful followers. His mother, and His several brothers were also among the blood-relations present at the feast.

His appearance caused much interest and comment among the other guests. To some He was simply a traveling religious teacher, not uncommon in that land, to others He was an inspired prophet, bringing a wonderful Message to the Jewish people, as He had to the Persians, Egyptians and Hindus; to others he was more than this, and whispers of "He is the Messiah"; "The King of Israel," etc., began to circulate among those present, causing interest, uneasiness or disgust, according to the views of the hearers. But whenever He moved, He attracted attention by His manner, attitude and expression. All felt that here indeed was an Individual. Strange stories of His wanderings in strange lands added additional interest to His presence.

A feeling that something unusual was about to happen began to creep over the crowd, as is the case often preceding such events.

Mary, His mother, watched her son with longing eyes, for she saw that some strange change had come over Him, that was beyond her comprehension.

Toward the end of the feast, it began to be whispered around among the near relatives that the supply of wine was about exhausted, the attendance having been much greater than had been expected. This, to a Jewish family, was akin to a family disgrace, and anxious looks began to be exchanged among the members of the immediate family.

Tradition has it that Jesus was besought for aid by His mother and other female kinswoman. Just what they expected Him to do is not clear, but it is probable that they unconsciously recognized His greatness, and accorded Him the place of the natural Head of the Family, as being the most prominent member. At any rate, they asked His aid. What arguments they used, or what reasons they urged, we do not know, but whatever they were, they succeeded in winning Him to their side, and gaining from Him a promise of aid and assistance. But not until after He had remonstrated that these things were of no concern of His—that His powers were not to be trifled away in this manner. But His love for His mother, and His desire to reward her devotion and faith in Him, prevailed over the natural disinclination of the mystic to be a "wonder worker" and to exhibit his occult powers to grace a wedding-feast. He had long since learned the necessary but comparatively simple occult feat from His old Masters in far off India, that land of wonder-working. He knew that even the humbler Yogis of that land would smile at the working of such a simple miracle. And so the matter seemed to Him to be of but slight moment, and not as a prostitution of some of the higher occult powers. And feeling thus, He yielded to their requests for aid.

Then moving toward the court in which were stored a number of great jars of water, he fixed a keen, burning glance upon them, one by one, passing His hand rapidly over them, in a quick succession, He made the Mental Image that precedes all such manifestations of occult power, and then manifesting His power by using His Will in the manner known to all advanced occultists, He rapidly materialized the elements of the wine in the water, within the jars, and lo! the "miracle" had been wrought.

A wave of excitement passed over the crowded house. The guests flocked around the jars to taste of the wine that had been produced by occult power. The priests frowned their displeasure, and the authorities sneered and whispered "charlatan"; "fraud"; "shameful imposture"; and other expressions that always follow an occurrence of this kind.

Jesus turned away, in grief and sorrow. Among the Hindus such a simple occult occurrence would have caused but little comment, while here among His own people it was considered to be a wonderful miracle by some, while others regarded it as a trick of a traveling conjurer and charlatan.

What manner of people were these to whom He had decided to deliver the Message of Life? And, sighing deeply, He passed from the house, and returned to His camp.

THE FIFTH LESSON

THE FOUNDATION OF THE WORK

There is but an imperfect record in the Gospels of the first year of Jesus' ministry among the Jews. Theologians have spoken of it as the "Year of Obscurity," but the Occult traditions speak of it as a most important year of His ministry, for in it He laid firm foundations for His future work.

He travelled all over the country, establishing little circles of disciples and centres of interest. In cities, towns, villages and hamlets, He left behind Him little bands of faithful students who kept alive the flame of Truth, which steadily kindled the lamps of others who were attracted by the light. Always among the humblest He labored, seemingly impressed with the idea that the work must be begun on the lowest rounds of society's ladder. But after a while a few of the more pretentious people began to attend the meetings, often brought there by curiosity. They came to smile and be amused, but many were impressed and remained to pray. The leaven had been well mixed in the loaf of Jewish society and it was beginning to work.

Once more the season of the Feast of the Passover arrived and found Jesus with His followers in Jerusalem and in the Temple. What memories the scene awakened in His mind. He could see the same scenes in which He had participated seventeen years before. Once more He saw the pitiful slaughter of the innocent lambs, and witnessed the flow of the sacrificed blood over the altars and the stones of the floor of the courts. Once more He saw the senseless mummery of the priestly ceremonies, which seemed more pitiful than ever to His developed mind. He knew that His vision had shown that He was to be slaughtered even as the sacrificial lambs, and there arose in His mind that comparison which stayed with Him ever after—that picture of Himself as the Lamb sacrificed on the Altar of Humanity. As pure as was this figure in His mind, it seems pitiful that in the centuries to come His followers would fall into the error (as equally cruel as that of the Hebrews) of imagining that His death was a sacrifice demanded by a cruel Deity to satisfy the Divine Wrath which had been kindled by the sight of Man's shortcomings and sins. The barbarous conception of a wrathful God whose anger against His people could be appeased only by the bloody slaughter of innocent creatures, is fully equalled by the theological dogmas that the same Divine Wrath could be, and was, appeased by the blood of Jesus, the Master who had come to deliver the Message of Truth. Such a conception is worthy of only the most barbarous and primitive minds. And yet it has been preached and taught for centuries—in the very name of Jesus Himself—and men have been persecuted and put to death because they refused to believe that the Supreme Creator of the Universe could be such a malignant, cruel, revengeful Being, or that the One Mind of All could be flattered and cajoled into forgiveness by the sight of the death of the Man of Sorrows. It seems almost incredible that such a teaching could have arisen from the pure teachings of Jesus, and that such has been Man's incapacity to grasp the Inner Teachings, that the Church built upon Jesus' ministry has adopted and insisted upon the acceptance of such dogmas. But this baneful cloud of ignorance and barbaric thought is gradually lifting, until even now the intelligent minds in the Church refuse to accept or teach the doctrine in its original crudity, they either passing it over in silence, or else dressing it in a more attractive garb.

Jesus taught no such barbarous things. His conception of Deity was of the highest, for He had received the most advanced teachings of the Mystics, who had instructed Him in the Mystery of the Immanent God, abiding everywhere and in all things. He had advanced far beyond the conception of Deity which pictured the One as a savage, bloodthirsty, vengeful, hating, tribal deity, ever crying for sacrifices and burnt-offerings, and capable of the meanest of human emotions. He saw this conception as He saw the conception of other races and peoples, all of which had their tribal or national gods, which loved that particular tribe or people, and which hated all other races or nationalities. He saw that back of, and behind, all these barbarous and primitive conceptions of Deity there dwelt an ever calm and serene Being, the Creator and Ruler of countless Universes—millions and millions of worlds—filling all space, and above all of the petty attributes that had been bestowed upon the petty gods of human creation. He knew that the God of each nation, of each person in fact, was but a magnified idea of the characteristics of the nation or individual in question. And he knew that Hebrew conception was no exception to this rule.

To anyone having grown to an appreciation of the grandeur and greatness of the idea of an Immanent Universal Being, the dogma of a Deity demanding a blood sacrifice to appease its wrath is too pitiful and degrading to be worth even a moment's serious consideration. And to such a one the prostitution of the high teachings of Jesus by the introduction of such a base conception is a source of righteous indignation and earnest protest. The Mystics in the Christian Church throughout the centuries have never accepted any such teachings, although the persecution of the church authorities have prevented their protests being made openly until of late years. The Mystics alone have kept alive the Light of the Truth through the Dark Ages of the Christian Church. But now has come the dawn of a new day, and the Church itself is seeing the Light, and the pulpits are beginning to resound with the truth of Mystic Christianity. And in the years to come the Teachings of Jesus, the Master, will flow pure and clear, once more freed from the corrupting dogmas which so long polluted the Fount.

As Jesus wandered silently through the courts and chambers of the Temple, His indignation was aroused by a sight which seemed to Him to portray more forcibly than aught else the degradation which had fallen upon the Temple by reason of the corruption of the priesthood. Grouped around the steps and outer courts of the Temple He saw the groups of brokers, money-changers and merchants who were doing a thriving business with the thousands of strangers attending the Feast. The money-changers were exchanging the coins of the realm for the inferior coins of the outlying regions, charging a large commission for the exchange. The brokers were buying articles, or loaning money on them, from the poor pilgrims, who were sacrificing their personal belongings for cash with which they might purchase the animals for the sacrifice. The merchants had droves of cattle, flocks of sheep and cages of doves within the sacred precincts of the Temple, which they were selling to the pilgrims who wished to offer sacrifices. Tradition has it that the corrupt priesthood profited by the sale of these "privileges" granted to this horde of traffickers in the Temple precincts. The vile practice had gradually crept in and established a firm foothold in the Temple, although contrary to the ancient practice.

To Jesus the horrible scenes of the Temple sacrificial rites seemed to focus in this final exhibition of greed, materialism and lack of spirituality. It seemed to be blasphemy and sacrilege of the most glaring type. And His very soul felt nauseated and outraged by the sight. His fingers twitched, and laying hold of a bundle of knotted cords which had been used by some cattle-driver to urge forward his herd, He rushed forward upon the horde of traffickers, whirling His instrument of chastisement over the shoulders and backs of the offenders, driving them out in a frantic rout, upsetting their benches and paraphernalia, crying in a voice of authority,

"Out, ye wretches! This is the House of the Lord, and ye have made it a den of thieves." The "Meek and lowly Nazarene" became an avenger of the prostitution of the Temple.

The brokers, money-changers and merchants fled before His mighty charge, leaving their scattered money over the floors of the Temple. They dared not return, for Jesus had aroused the wrath of the people against them, and a cry arose for the old practice of protecting the sacred place against such invasion. But the traffickers sought out the High-priests and complained bitterly of this annulment of their "privileges" and "franchises," for which they had paid so highly. And the High-priests, being compelled to refund the price paid for the concessions, were much wrought up over the matter, and then and there swore vengeance against the Master who had dared interfere with their system of what the world now calls by the suggestive name of "graft." And this vengeance and hatred waxed stronger each moment, and was to a great extent the moving factor in the schemes and intrigues which two years later resulted in the frightful scene on Calvary.

The succeeding months were filled with wanderings up and down the land, spreading the work and making new converts and followers. Jesus did not take the position of a great preacher at this time, but seemed to be rather a teacher of the few whom He gathered around Him at each point and place. He observed but few ceremonies, that of Baptism being the principal one, and which, as we have shown, was an Essenic rite having an occult and mystical significance. The students of the New Testament may read between its leaves the history of the ministry of Jesus at this time, noting the working of the leaven in the mass of the Jewish mind.

About this time Jesus was sorely distressed at the terrible news which reached Him regarding the fate of his cousin, John the Baptist, who had been His Forerunner. The Baptist had dared to thrust his preachings and rebukes into the very precincts of a corrupt court, and had brought down upon his head the natural consequences of his rashness. Herod had thrust him into a gloomy dungeon and there were rumors of a worse fate yet in store for him. And that fate soon overtook him. Refusing the chance of life and liberty that was promised him if he would but break his vows of asceticism and indulge the passionate desires of a royal princess,— turning away from the base proposal with the horror of the true mystic,—he met his fate like a man knowing the Truth, and the head which graced the royal platter bore upon its face no expression of fear or regret. John had conquered even in Death.

Jesus retired once more into the Desert upon the news of John's death reaching him. Added to His sorrow came the conviction that there was a new work set before Him to do. John's death necessitated a combining of the work of the Baptist with that of Jesus' own ministry. The followers of the two teachers must be combined into one great body, under the supervision of the Master Himself, aided by the most worthy and capable of His disciples. The tragic death of John played a most important part in the future ministry of the Master, and He sought the solace and inspiration of the Desert in His consideration of the plans and details of His new work. Students will note that from the time He emerged from the Desert He threw off the cloak of reserve and retirement and stepped boldly before the people as an ardent preacher to multitudes and an impassioned orator and public speaker. No more the little circle of appreciative students—the rostrum with the great crowds of hearers were His from that time.

Returning from His work in Samaria and Judea, He once more made Galilee the scene of His principal work. The new spirit which He now threw into His preaching attracted the attention of the public, and enormous crowds attended His meetings. He spoke now with a new air of authority, differing greatly from His former mild tones as a teacher of the few. Parables and allegories and other rich Oriental figures of speech fell from His lips, and many of the educated classes flocked to hear the wonderful young orator and preacher. He seemed to have an intuitive insight into the minds of His hearers, and His appeals reached their hearts as personal calls to righteousness, right thinking and right living. From this time on His ministry assumed the character of an active propaganda, instead of the usual quiet mission of the Mystic.

And here began that remarkable series of wonder workings or "miracles" which He evidently employed to attract the attention of the public and at the same time to perform kindly and worthy acts. Not that He used these wonder-workings as a bid for sensational interest or self-glory—the character of Jesus rendered such a course impossible—but He knew that nothing would so attract the interest of an Oriental race as occurrences of this kind, and He hoped to then awaken in them a real spiritual interest and fervor, which would rise far above the demand for "miracles." In adopting this course Jesus followed the example of the holy men in India, with whose works He was personally familiar, owing to His sojourn in that land.

And, then let us say, that advanced occultists see nothing

"supernatural" nor incredible in these "miracles" of Jesus. On the contrary, they know them to be the result of the application of certain well established natural laws, which, while almost unknown to the masses of people, are still known and occasionally made use of by the advanced occultists of all lands. Skeptics and unbelievers may sneer at these things, and many faint-faith Christians may wish to apologize or "explain" these wonderful happenings, but the advanced occultist needs no "explanations" nor apologies. He has more faith than the church-goer, for he knows of the existence and use of these occult powers latent in Man. There is no material effect or phenomenon that is "supernatural"—the Laws of Nature are in full operation on the material plane and cannot be overcome. But there are among such Natural Laws certain phases and principles that are so little known to the average mind that when they are manifested Nature's Laws seemed to be transcended, and the result is called "a miracle." The occult tradition tells us that Jesus was a past-master in the knowledge and application of the occult forces of nature, and that even the wonders that He wrought during His Jewish ministry were but as child's play when compared with those that He might have manifested had He seen fit to do so. In fact, it is believed that some of His greatest wonder-workings have never been recorded, for He always impressed upon His chosen followers the advisability of refraining from laying too much stress on these things. The "miracles" recorded in the Gospels were only those which were most widely known among the people. The greater-wonders were deemed too sacred for common gossip.

When the Master and His followers reached Cana, which, by the way, had been the scene of his first "miracle"—the changing of the water into wine at the wedding feast—one of the most striking of His earlier manifestations of occult power occurred. An influential citizen of Capernaum, a town a score of miles distant, who met Him and besought His aid and power in the interest of his young son, who lay dying at his home. The man besought Jesus to hasten to Capernaum to heal the youth ere he die. Jesus smiled kindly upon him and bade him return to his son, for the youth was even now restored to health and strength and life. His hearers were astounded at the reply and the doubters smiled knowingly, foreseeing a defeat for the young Master when the news of the youth's death should become known. Those of His followers who were faint of heart and weak of faith felt most uncomfortable and began to whisper the "if" of doubt. But Jesus continued His working with a calm air of certainty, without further remarks. It was the seventh hour of the day when the words were spoken.

The father hastened homeward to see whether the Master had succeeded or failed. A day or two passed with no word from Capernaum. The scoffers of the wedding feast repeated their sneers and revilings—the word "charlatan" was again heard passing from lip to lip. Then came news from the distant village, and upon its arrival the voice of scorn was stilled, and the hearts of the faint again beat freely. The word came that when the father had reached his house he was greeted by the household with cries of joy and news that at the seventh hour the fever had abated and the crisis had been passed.

And yet the "miracle" above recorded was no greater than many occultists have performed in all times—no greater than the many similar cures that have been performed by the modern healers of the many metaphysical cults. It was simply an application of the subtle forces of nature called into operation by mental concentration. It was an instance of what in modern phrase is called "absent treatment" along metaphysical lines. In saying this we wish in no way to detract from the wonder that Jesus had wrought, but merely to let the student know that the power is still possessed by others and is not a "supernatural" thing but the operation of purely natural laws.

About this time there occurred another event in His life, and a manifestation of His power which is noted in the New Testament and which is told in the occult tradition with somewhat more detail. It occurred when Jesus visited his home town of Nazareth on the eve of the Jewish Sabbath. He rested over night and then the following morning betook Himself to the regular services in the local synagogue. He took the seat which He had occupied as a young boy with Joseph. No doubt the familiar scene awakened memories of His strange youthful history in His mind. Then, much to His surprise, He heard Himself called to the platform to conduct the service. It must be remembered that Jesus was a regular rabbi, or priest, by birth, education and training, and was entitled to Conduct the Jewish service. No doubt His townspeople wished to hear their young townsman address and exhort them. He took the place of authority in the synagogue and proceeded to read the regular service in the accustomed manner, as prescribed by the custom and laws of the church. The prayers, chantings and readings succeeded each other in their regular order. Then came the preaching of the sermon. Taking the sacred roll from its receptacle, He read the text from Isaiah, "The spirit of the Lord is upon me because He hath anointed me to preach the good tidings," etc. Then He began his exposition of the text He had just read.

But instead of the expected customary words and illustrations—technical theological hair-splitting and dreary platitudes—He began to preach in a manner unknown to the Nazarenes. His opening sentence broke the silence and greatly startled and disturbed the congregation. "This day is this Scripture fulfilled in your ears," were his opening words. And then He began a statement of His conception of His ministry and His Message. Thrusting aside all precedent and musty authority, He boldly proclaimed that He had come to establish a new conception of the Truth—a conception that would overturn the priestly policy of formalism and lack of spirituality—a conception that would ignore forms and ceremonies, and cleave close to the spirit of the Sacred Teachings. And then He began a scathing denunciation of the lack of spiritual advancement among the Jewish people—their materialism and desire for physical enjoyments and their drifting away from the highest ideals of the race. He preached the mystic doctrine, and insisted that they be applied to the problems of everyday life and conduct. He brought down the teachings of the Kaballah from the cloudy heights, and set them before the people in plain, practical form. He bade them aspire to great spiritual heights, forsaking the base ideals to which they had clung. He ran counter to every custom and prejudice of the people before Him, and showed a lack of reverence for all of their petty forms and traditions. He bade them leave the illusions of material life and follow the Light of the Spirit wherever it might lead them. These and many other things told He them.

And then arose a disturbance among the congregation. They began to interrupt and question Him, and many were the contradictions and denials hurled at Him from the benches. Some began to sneer at His pretensions as the Bearer of the Message, and demanded that He work a wonder or "miracle" and give them a sign. This demand He flatly refused to grant, not deeming the same proper, or in accordance with the occult custom which always frowned upon wonder-working in response to such a demand. Then they began to abuse Him and cries of "charlatan" and "fraud" began to resound from the walls of the synagogue. They reminded Him of His humble birth and condition of His parents, and refused to believe that any such person as He had any right to claim extraordinary powers or privileges. Then came from His lips the famous saying, "A prophet is not without honor, save in his own country."

Then He began a fresh assault upon their prejudices and

narrow views—their pet superstitions and bigotry. He stripped from them their garb of hypocrisy and assumed piety, and showed them their naked souls in all their ugliness and moral uncleanliness. He poured burning invective and vitriolic denunciations into their midst, and spared no terms that could properly be applied to them. In a short time the congregation was beside itself with rage, and the pretended righteous indignation of a flock of hypocrites and formalists who had heard themselves described in disrespectful terms by one they regarded as an upstart young man from the lower classes of their virtuous community. They felt that they had bestowed a flattering honor upon Him, as a mark of consideration for a young townsman upon His return from a foreign and domestic missionary tour. And now to think that He had thus basely betrayed their courtesy and showed in how little esteem He really held them—surely this was beyond human endurance. And then the storm broke upon Him.

Leaving their seats in the synagogue, the congregation rushed upon the young preacher, and tearing Him from the platform, they pushed Him out of the building. And then the jostling, hustling, pushing crowd carried Him before them along the village streets and out into the suburbs. He resisted not, deeming it unworthy to struggle with them. At last, however, He was compelled to defend Himself. He perceived that it was the intention of the mob to push Him over a precipice that had been formed on the side of a hill just beyond the town limits. He waited patiently until they had urged Him to the very brink of the decline, and until it needed but one strong push to press Him over its edge and into the gorge below. And then He exerted His occult forces in a proper self-defense. Not a blow struck He—not a man did He smite with the wondrous occult power at His command, which would have paralyzed their muscles or even have stretched them lifeless at His feet. No, he controlled Himself with a firm hand, and merely bent upon them a look. But such a look!

A glance in which was concentrated the mighty Will developed by mystic knowledge and occult practice. It was the Gaze of the Occult Master, the power of which ordinary men may not withstand. And the mob, feeling its mighty force, experienced the sensation of abject fear and terror. Their hair arose, their eyes started from their sockets, their knees shook under them, and then, with a wild shout of horror they began to scatter and fly, making a wide pathway for the Man of Mystery who now strode through their ranks with that awful gaze which seemed to pierce the veil of mortality and to peer at things ineffable and beyond human ken. And with His eyes refusing to look again upon the familiar scenes of His youth, He departed from Nazareth, forsaking it forever as His home place. Verily, indeed, the Prophet hath no honor in His own land. Those who should have been His staunchest supporters were the first in His own land to threaten Him with violence. The attempt of Nazareth was the prophecy of Calvary, and Jesus so knew it. But He had set his feet upon The Path, and drew not back from it.

Turning His back upon Nazareth, Jesus established a new centre or home in Capernaum, which place remained the nearest approach to home to Him during the remainder of His Ministry and until His death. The traditions have it that His mother came to live also at Capernaum, together with some of His brothers. It is also related that his sisters and brothers, both those remaining at Nazareth and those removing to Capernaum, were sorely vexed with Him at His conduct at the synagogue, which they deemed not "respectable" nor proper, and they accordingly looked upon Him as an eccentric relative whose vagaries had brought disrepute upon the family. He was regarded much in the light of a "black-sheep" and "undesirable relation" by all of His family except His mother, who still clung to her beloved first-born. The mother made her home with some of the brothers and sisters of Jesus, but He was not made welcome there, but was looked upon as an outcast and wanderer. He once spoke of this, saying that while the birds and beasts had nests and homes, He, the Son of Man, had nowhere to lay his head. And so He wandered around in His own land, as He had in foreign countries, an ascetic, living upon the alms of the people who loved Him and listened to His words. And in so doing He followed the plans and life of the Hindu ascetics, who even unto this day so live, "with yellow-robe and begging bowl," and "without money or scrip in their purses." The Jewish ascetic—for such was Jesus—has His counterparts in the wandering holy-men of India and Persia today.

But it must be remembered that even in Jesus' time, the spectacle of a rabbi living this ascetic life, forsaking the emoluments of His priestly rank and deliberately taking up the roll of a poverty-stricken mendicant, was a rare one. It ran contrary to all the thrifty and prudent customs and ideals of the race. It was an importation from the Essenes, or from the strange people of far-off lands, and it was not relished by the Jewish authorities, or people who preferred the synagogues and Temple, with their sleek, well-fed priests, with fancy robes and attractive ceremonies.

Making His base at Capernaum, Jesus began to form His band

of disciples with more show of a working organization. To some He delegated certain authority, and bade them perform certain dues of the ministry. For some reason He selected some of His leading lieutenants from the ranks of the fishermen who plied their vocation along the waters of that port of the country. The fishers of fish became the fishers of men. Jesus became very popular among the fishing fraternity, and the legends, as well as the New Testament narratives, tell of instances in which He bade His poor fishermen friends (who had been unfortunate in their day's haul) to let down their nets at some point indicated by Him, when to their surprise and joy their nets would be filled to overflowing.

Little acts of kindness bestowed here and there among the humbler classes tended to have Jesus looked upon and spoken of as a friend of the people, but which reputation excited the jealousy of the authorities who held that such acts could be prompted by none other than a selfish motive, and that motive the incitement of the masses to rebellion in the interest of Himself as a Messiah. And so, we see His very acts of kindness and compassion served to increase the suspicion and hatred which the authorities, both ecclesiastical and temporal, had always felt toward Him.

His desire to alleviate the sufferings of the poor and wretched took Him much among these people and away from the so-called higher classes. The "plain people" were regarded by Him as the salt of the earth, and they, in turn, regarded Him as their champion and advisor. And especially to the sick did He devote His time and powers. He made many marvellous cures, a few only of which were recorded in the New Testament narratives. The occult legends state that these cures were of daily occurrence and that wherever He went He left behind Him a trail of people healed of all kinds of disorders, and that people flocked for miles to be healed of their infirmities. The Gospels relate that He cured great numbers of people by the simple process of laying on of hands (a favorite method of occult healers) "he laid his hands on every one of them and healed them."

It is related that at Capernaum his attention was directed toward a madman, who suddenly cried out, "I know Thee, Thou Holy One of God," whereupon Jesus spoke a few authoritative words and cured him of his malady, by methods that will describe the nature of the man's psychic disturbance to any advanced student of occultism. Demoniac possession is not believed in by orthodox Christians of today, but Jesus evidently shared the belief in obsession held by students of Psychism and similar subjects, judging from the words He used in relieving this man from his malady. We advise our students to read the Gospel records in connection with these lessons, in order to follow the subject along the old familiar paths, but with the additional light of the interpretation of Mystic Christianity.

The growing reputation of Jesus as a healer of the sick soon taxed His physical powers to the utmost. He felt Himself called upon to do the work of a dozen men, and His nature rebelled at the unequal task imposed upon it. It seemed as if all Capernaum were sick. Her streets were crowded by seekers after health and strength. At last He perceived that His work as a Teacher was being submerged in His work as a Healer. And, after a period of prayer and meditation, He put aside from Him the claims of humanity for the healing of physical ills, and turning His back upon the waiting patients at Capernaum, He once more started forward on His pilgrimage as a Preacher of the Message, and thereafter would heal physical ills only occasionally, and, instead, devote the main portion of His time to preaching the Truth to those who were ready to hear it. It was a hard thing for a man with the tender heart of Jesus to leave behind Him the crowd of patients at Capernaum, but it was necessary for Him to do so, else He would have remained merely an occult healer of physical ailments instead of the Messenger of the Truth whose work it was to kindle in many places the Flame of the Spirit, that would serve as the true Light of the World long after the physical bodies of all then living had been again resolved to dust.

And so, leaving behind Him Capernaum and its wailing multitudes, He, followed by His disciples, moved out toward the open country, to spread the glad tidings and to bring to the hearts of many "that peace which passeth all understanding."

THE SIXTH LESSON

THE WORK OF ORGANIZATION

Leaving Capernaum behind Him, with its crowds of invalids seeking healing, and fighting off the demands that would have rendered Him a professional healer instead of a Teacher and preacher of the Message of Truth, Jesus passed on to other parts of the land, taking with Him the band of disciples and faithful followers who now traveled with Him.

But He did not altogether relinquish His healing work. He merely made it an incident of His ministry, and did not allow it to interfere with His preaching and teaching. The Gospel narratives show a number of remarkable cures made by Him at this time, and the few recorded cases are, of course, merely occasional incidents that stand out in the minds of the people among hundreds of less noticeable cases.

The cure of the leper is one of such remarkable cases. Leprosy was a foul disease much dreaded by the people of Oriental countries. And the unfortunate person afflicted by it became an outcast and pariah from whom all others fled as from an unclean and impure thing.

There was a leper in the part of the country in which Jesus was traveling and teaching. He heard of the wonderful gift of healing accredited to the young preacher, and he determined to get into His presence and beg His aid. How the leper managed to get through the crowds and into the presence of Jesus is not known, but it must have required great strategy on his part, for such people were not permitted to pass in and among crowds of other people. But in some way the leper contrived to come face to face with Jesus as the latter walked alone in meditation, away from his followers.

The loathsome creature raised its repulsive form, the picture of human misery and woe, and confronting the Master, demanded from Him the exercise of the Gift of Healing. No doubt of His power was in the leper's mind—his face shone with faith and expectation. Jesus gazed earnestly into the distorted features that shone with the fire of a fervent faith such as is rarely seen on the face of man, and touched with this testimony to His power and motives, He moved toward the leper, defying the laws of the country, which forbade the same. Not only this, but He even laid His hands upon the unclean flesh, defying all the laws of reason in so doing, and fearlessly passed His hand over the leper's face, crying aloud, "Be thou clean!"

The leper felt a strange thrill running through his veins and over his nerves, and every atom of his body seemed to be tingling with a peculiar burning and smarting sensation. Even as he looked he saw the color of his flesh changing and taking on the hue of the flesh of the healthy person. The numbness departed from the affected portion of his body, and he could actually feel the thrill and tingle of the life currents that were at work with incredible speed building up new cells, tissue and muscle. And still Jesus held His hands against the flesh of the leper, allowing the life current of highly vitalized prana to pour from His organism into that of the leper, just as a storage battery of great power replenishes and recharges an electrical appliance. And back of it all was the most potent, trained Will of the Master Occultist directing the work.

And then He bade the healed man depart and comply with the laws regarding purification and change of garments, including the appearance before the priests to receive a certificate of cleanliness. And He also bade him that nothing should be said regarding the nature or particulars of the cure. For some good reason He wished to escape the notoriety or fame that the report of such a wonderful cure would be sure to excite.

But alas! this was asking too much of human nature, and the healed leper, running with great leaps and bounds, began shouting and crying aloud the glad tidings of his marvelous cure, that all men might know what a great blessing had come to him. In spite of the injunction laid upon him, he began to sing aloud the praises of the Master who had manifested such an unheard-of power over the foul disease that had held him in its grasp until a few hours before. With wild gestures and gleaming eyes he told the story again and again, and it was taken up and repeated from person to person, until the whole town and countryside were familiar with the great news. Imagine such an event occurring in a small country town in our own land today, and you will realize what an excitement must have been occasioned in that home place of the leper.

And then occurred that which Jesus had doubtless seen when He forbade the leper to repeat the news of the cure. The whole region became excited and immense crowds gathered around Him and His disciples, crying aloud for new wonders and miracles. The curious sensation-seekers were there in full force, crowding out those whom He wished to reach by His teachings. And more than this, great numbers of sick and crippled people crowded around Him crying for aid and cure. The scenes of Capernaum were repeated. Even the lepers began flocking in, in defiance of law and custom, and the authorities were beside themselves with anger and annoyance. Not only the temporal authorities and the priests were arrayed against Him, as of old, but now He managed to arouse the opposition of the physicians of those days, who saw their practice ruined by this man whom they called a charlatan and deceiver threatening and destroying the health of the people, whose physical welfare was safe only in their (the physicians') hands and keeping.

And so Jesus was compelled to close His ministry at this place and move on to another village.

Another case which attracted much attention was that which occurred in Galilee when He was preaching in a house. In the midst of His discourse both He and His audience were startled by the sight of a figure on a bed being lowered down among the crowd of listeners from the roof surrounding the open court in the center of the house. It was a poor paralyzed man whom friends had contrived to hoist up and then lower down before Jesus in such a manner as could not escape the attention of the Master. It is related that the piteous appeal of the sufferer, and the faith which had inspired such great energy on the part of his friends, attracted the interest and sympathy of Jesus, and He paused in His discourse and made another of those instantaneous cures which are possible only to the most advanced adepts in the science of spiritual healing.

Then came the scene of the Wells of Bethesda—a region abounding in "healing waters" to which the sick and afflicted came to regain their health. The crowds of sick were being carried to the springs by friends or paid attendants, who pushed aside the weaker ones and fought their way to the wells. Jesus walked among the crowds, and at last His attention was attracted toward a poor fellow who lay upon his cot away off from the waters. He had no friends to carry him nearer, nor money for paid attendants. And he had not strength enough to crawl there himself. He filled the air with his moans and cries and bewailings of his unfortunate lot. Jesus walked up to him, and holding his attention by a firm look of authority and power, cried to him suddenly in a voice that demanded obedience, "Take up thy bed and walk!" The man, startled into obedience, did as directed, and much to his surprise, and that of the crowd gathered around, found that he was able to move about freely—a well man.

This cure also aroused not only the greatest interest but also the antagonism of the ecclesiastical authorities. It appears that the cure had been made on the Sabbath day, and that it was against the ecclesiastical law to heal the sick in any way upon that day; and also that the patient had performed manual work on the Sabbath in carrying his bed upon the orders of the Healer. And the good pious folk, urged on by the priests, began to abuse and condemn the Healer and patient, after the manner of the formal pietists of all lands and times, even of our own. Clinging to the letter of the law, these people overlook its spirit—bound by the forms, they fail to see the meaning lying back of all forms and ceremonies.

Braving the storm that was arising around Him, Jesus boldly walked to the Temple. He was plunged in a sea of conflicting opinions and voices. On the one hand was the healed man and those who sympathized with him, in earnest argument concerning the righteousness of the deed. But arrayed against these few were the good folk of the place who loudly denounced the Sabbath-breaker and demanded His punishment. Were the ancient laws of Moses to be thus defied by this presumptuous Nazarene, whose religious ideas were sadly lacking in orthodoxy? Surely not! Punish the upstart! And again Jesus was in actual peril of bodily hurt, or perhaps even death, owing to the religious bigotry of the orthodox people.

Jesus was ever a foe to the stupid formalism and ignorant fanaticism regarding "holy days," which is ever a characteristic of certain classes of mind among people. On the above occasion, as well as upon other occasions, and notably upon the occasion of the Sabbath when He directed His hungry disciples to pick corn to satisfy their hunger, Jesus opposed the strict, ironclad law of Sabbath observance. He was ever filled with the idea that the "Sabbath was made for man, and not man for the Sabbath." There was nothing Puritanical about the Master, and in view of His attitude regarding this matter it is surprising to witness the attitude of some in our own time who, wearing His livery, oppose these teachings of His in theory and practice.

And so, driven out once more by the intolerance and bigotry of the public, Jesus returned again to Galilee, His land of retreat and rest, and the scene of much of His best work. Galilee was filled with His many followers and admirers, and He was less in danger of disturbance and persecution there than in the neighborhood of Jerusalem. Large congregations attended His ministry there, and His converts were numbered by the thousand. The village contained many persons healed by His power, and His name was a household word.

And upon His return He entered into a new stage of His work. He had decided to divide His ministry among His twelve most advanced disciples, as it had now reached proportions beyond His ability to personally control. And, as was customary to Him upon all great occasions, He sought the solitudes for meditation and spiritual strength before finally investing His twelve Apostles with the high authority of their mission. He spent the night on one of the hills near Capernaum, from which He descended the following morning, wearied in body from want of rest, but strong in soul and spirit.

Then He gathered the Twelve around Him, and in a secret meeting divulged to them certain deep truths and secrets, adding certain instructions regarding healing work, and calling upon them for the highest allegiance to Him and His work.

The Gospel narratives have but very little to say regarding Jesus' work in the instruction of the Twelve for their future mission. And the average student of the narratives goes on without thinking of the marvelous mental and spiritual development that must have been manifested by the Apostles during their transition from humble fishermen, and men of similar vocations, to highly developed teachers of advanced spiritual truths. To the occultist especially this ordinary view seems astounding, for he realizes the many arduous steps necessary to be trodden by the feet of the Neophyte before he becomes an Initiate, and the higher steps awaiting the Initiate before he may become a Master. And such a one realizes the mighty task that Jesus performed in developing and unfolding the spiritual natures of such a body of men until they become worthy to be His chosen representatives and teachers. The occult traditions have it that Jesus had pursued a systematic course of instruction of His chosen disciples, bringing them up rapidly through degree after degree of mystic attainment and occult knowledge, until finally they were ready for the finishing touches at His hands. And the occasion that we are now considering was the time when the final degrees were imparted to them.

It must be remembered that the Apostles were endowed with the mastery of the occult forces of nature which enabled them to perform the "miracles" of healing similar to those of Jesus. And it must not be supposed for a moment that an occult Master of so high a degree of attainment as that reached by Jesus would have allowed His disciples to use such mighty power without also instructing them fully in the nature of the forces they were using, and of the best methods of employing the same. And such knowledge could not be imparted without the fundamental truths of nature being understood by them, which understanding was possible only to those who had grasped the great Basic Truths of the Science of Being.

In short, the traditions are that the Twelve Apostles were gradually initiated into the great degrees of the Occult Brotherhoods of which and in which Jesus was a Master. He gathered together a great store of occult information and mystic lore, and condensing the same into a plain, practical, simple system, He imparted it fully and thoroughly to those whom He had elected to be His chief co-workers and His successors after His death, which He knew full well was not far off.

These facts must be fully understood by the student of Mystic Christianity who wishes to grasp the secret of the early Christian Church after the death of Christ. The wonderful headway manifested by the movement could not have been given by mere followers and believers in the Master. It usually follows that when the great head of an organization dies the movement disintegrates or loses power unless he has been able to "communicate his spirit" to some chosen followers. And this Jesus did. And it was only to men who thoroughly grasped the fundamental truths and principles of His teachings that such "spirit" could have been imparted.

There was an exoteric teaching for the multitude, and an esoteric teaching for the Twelve. There are many Scriptural passages which go to show this fact, which was well known to the early Fathers of the Church. And upon the occasion which we have mentioned the last great Basic Truths were explained to the Twelve, and from that time henceforward they were regarded and treated as Masters by Jesus, and not as mere students, as had been the case before that time. And arising from that final instruction came the Sermon of the Mount.

The Sermon of the Mount, that most wonderful and complete of any of the public utterances of Jesus, was delivered almost immediately after the Choosing of the Twelve Apostles. And it was intended even more for them than for the multitudes gathered around to hear His preaching. He knew that the Twelve could interpret it by reason of the Inner Teachings that they had received from Him. And almost forgetting the congregation gathered around and about Him, He elucidated the Inner teachings for the benefit of the Chosen Few.

The Sermon of the Mount can be understood only by means of the Master Key of the Inner Teachings, which opens the door of the mind to an understanding of the hard sayings and veiled mystic import of many of His precepts. We shall devote considerable space in one of our later lessons of this series to a consideration of the Inner Meaning of this great sermon and teaching, and therefore shall not go into details regarding it in the present lesson, deeming it better to proceed with the story of the Master's Work.

A few days after the delivery of the Sermon of the Mount, the Master left Capernaum and traveled from town to town visiting His various centers of teaching, as was His custom. On the journey Jesus performed a feat of occult power that proved Him to be one of the Highest Adepts of the Occult Brotherhoods, for to none other would such a manifestation have been possible. Even some of the highest Oriental Masters would have refused to undertake the task that He set before Himself to do.

The company was leisurely proceeding on its way, when nearing a small town they met a funeral procession coming in their direction. Preceded by the band of women chanting the mournful dirges according to the Galileean custom, the cortege slowly wended its way. The etiquette of the land required strangers to join in the mourning when they came in contact with a funeral procession, and the company assumed a mournful and respectful demeanor, and many joined in the dirge which was being chanted by the procession.

But Jesus invaded the privacy of the procession in a manner shocking to those who held closely to the familiar forms and customs. Stepping up to the bier, He stood in front of it and bade the carriers halt and set it down. A murmur of indignation ran through the ranks of the mourners, and some strode forward to rebuke the presumptuous stranger who dared to violate the dignity of the funeral in this way. But something in His face held them back. Then a strange feeling passed over the crowd. Jesus was known to a number of the mourners, and some of those who had witnessed some of His wonder-workings began to whisper that strange things were about to happen, and the ranks were broken as the people flocked around the Master at the bier.

The corpse was that of a young man, and his widowed mother stood beside the pale figure stretched upon the bier, and spreading her arms in front of it, she seemed to ward off the profaning touch of the strange man who confronted it. But the stranger looked upon her with a look of transcendent love, and in a voice vibrant with the tenderest feeling said unto her, "Mother, weep not—cease thy mourning." Amazed, but impressed, she turned an appealing gaze to Him who had thus bidden her. Her mother love and instinct caught a new expression in His eyes, and her heart bounded with a wonderful hope of something, she knew not what. What did the Nazarene mean? Her boy was dead, and even God Himself never disturbed the slumber of the body from which the spirit had flown. But still what meant that expression—why that leap and throbbing of her heart?

Then with a gesture of authority the Master caused the crowd to draw back from the bier, until at last there remained only the corpse, the mother and Himself in a cleared space in the center. Then a strange and wonderful scene began. With His gaze fixed upon the face of the corpse, and in an attitude that indicated a supreme effort of His will, the Master was seen to be making some mighty effort which called into play the highest forces at His command. The Apostles, having been instructed by Him in Occult power, recognized the nature of the manifestation, and their faces paled, for they knew that He was not only pouring out His vital force into the body in order to recharge it with prana, but that He was also essaying one of the highest and most difficult of occult feats—that of summoning back from the Astral Plane the higher vehicles and the Astral Body—the very soul of the youth—and forcing it once more into its mortal frame, which He had recharged with vital energy and strength. They knew that He, by the mightiest effort of His will, was reversing the process of death. And with a full appreciation of the real nature of the wonder that was being worked before them, their limbs trembled beneath them and their breath came from them in gasps.

Then cried the people, "What saith this man to the corpse?" "Arise, youth! Open thine eyes! Breathe freely! Arise, I say unto thee—arise!" Did this stranger dare to defy God's own decree?

The corpse opened its eyes and stared around in wild amaze, the glare not fully faded away! Its chest heaved in great agonizing gasps as if fighting again for life! Then its arms were lifted up—then its legs began to move—now it raised itself upright and began to babble meaningless words—now the look of recognition came into its eyes, and its arms clasped themselves around the mother's neck, while sob after sob broke from its lips! The dead lived—the corpse had come to life.

The people fell back overcome with the awful terror of the sight, and the funeral procession scattered in all directions, until only the sobbing mother and the youth remained, weeping in their mutual love and joy, and forgetting even the Master and His followers in their great flood of affection.

And, leaving them thus, Jesus and His followers passed away on their pilgrimage. But the fame of the miracle spread from town to town, even up to the great capital, Jerusalem. And men wondered or doubted, according to their natures, while the temporal and ecclesiastical authorities began to again ask themselves and each other whether this man were not a dangerous person and an enemy to established custom and order.

In one of His journeys Jesus found Himself invited to the house of a leading citizen of the town in which He was preaching. This citizen was one of the class known as Pharisees, whose characteristics were an extreme devotion and adherence to forms and ceremonies and a bigoted insistence upon the observance of the letter of the law. The Pharisees were the ultra-orthodox center of an orthodox people. They were the straight-laced brethren who walked so erect that they leaned backward. They were the people who thanked God that they were not like unto other men. They were the "uncommonly good" members of church and society. The very name stands even unto this day as a synonym for "pious sham."

Just why this Pharisee had invited the Master to dine with him is not easily understood. It is likely that it was a combination of curiosity and a desire to entrap his guest into statements and admissions that might be used against him. At any rate, the invitation was given and accepted.

The Master noted that certain little ceremonies usually extended by the Hebrews to a guest of equal standing were omitted by His host. His head was not anointed with the ceremonial oil, as was the custom in houses of this character when the guest was honored as an equal or desirable addition to the family gathering. Clearly He was regarded as a curiosity or "freak" rather than as a friend, and had been invited in such a spirit. But He said nothing, and passed over the slight. And the meal passed along smoothly up to a certain point.

The host and his guests were reclining easily, after the Oriental fashion, discussing various topics, when a woman pressed her way into the banquet hall. Her dress proclaimed her to be one of the women of easy virtue abounding in all Oriental towns. She was clad in showy apparel and her hair fell loosely over her shoulders after the custom of the women of her kind in that land. She fixed her eyes upon the Master and moved slowly toward him, much to the annoyance of the host, who feared a scene, for the Master would most likely administer a rebuke to the woman for presuming to intrude upon the presence of Him, a spiritual teacher.

But the woman still pressed forward toward Him, and at last, bending down low, her head touching His feet, she burst into tears. She had heard the Master preach some time before, and the seeds of

His teaching had taken root and had now blossomed within her heart; and she had come to acknowledge her allegiance and to render an offering to Him whom she revered. The coming into His presence was her token of a spiritual regeneration and a desire to begin a new life. Her tears flowed over His feet, and she dried them off with her long hair. Then she kissed His feet, as a token of her allegiance and worship.

From her neck hung a chain holding a little box filled with precious perfumed oil, which she esteemed highly, as did all the people of her race. The oil was of the nature of attar of roses and was the essential oil extracted from fragrant blossoms. She broke the seal and poured the fragrant oil over the hands and feet of the Master, who rebuked her not, but who accepted the tribute even from such a source. The host began to indulge in thoughts not flattering to the intelligence of his guest, and a scarcely concealed sneer appeared on his lips.

Then Jesus turned to His host and with a smile said to him: "Simon, in thy mind thou thinkest these words: 'If this man be indeed a prophet, would he not know what manner of woman this be who toucheth him, and would he not rebuke her and drive her from him?'" And the Pharisee was sorely confused, for the Master had read his thought word for word by the method known to occultists as telepathy. And then in gentle raillery the Master called his host's attention to the fact that the woman had performed the service which he, the host, had neglected to observe. Had she not bathed and dried His feet, as the Pharisee would have done had his guest been deemed worthy of honor? Had she not anointed Him with precious oil, as the host would have anointed an honored guest? Had she not impressed upon even His feet the kiss that etiquette required the host to impress upon the cheek of the esteemed visitor to his house? And as for the character of the woman, it had been fully recognized and forgiven. "Much hath been forgiven her, for she hath loved greatly." And, turning to the woman, He added, "Go in peace, for thy sins are forgiven thee." And the woman departed with a new expression on her face and a firm resolve in her heart, for the Master had forgiven and blessed her.

But by this act Jesus brought upon His head the hatred of the Pharisee and his friends. He had dared rebuke the host in his own palace, and had moreover arrogated to Himself the sacred rite to pronounce remission of sins, a right vested solely in the high-priest of the Temple, upon the performance of certain ceremonies and sacrifices upon the altar. He had flung defiance at vested ecclesiastical right and functions, even in the house of one of the stanchest adherents of formalism and authority—a Pharisee.

In this incident was shown not only the broadness of Jesus' views and the universality of His love, as well as His courage in defying the hated formalism, even in the palace of its stanchest advocates, but also His attitude toward women. The Jews as a race held women in but scant esteem. They were not deemed worthy to sit with the men in the synagogue. It was deemed unworthy of a man to mention his female relations in general company. They were regarded as inferior in every way to men, and were treated as almost unclean in their most sacred natural functions.

Toward fallen women especially Jesus was ever considerate. He saw their temptation and the social cruelty of their position. He resented "the double standard" of virtue which allowed a man to commit certain offenses and still be respected, while the woman who committed the same offense was damned socially, reviled and treated as a shameful outcast. He was ever ready to voice a defense for women of this kind, and seemed to be ever actuated by the sense of injustice in the attitude of men toward them, which finally voiced itself on a notable occasion when called upon to pass judgment upon the woman taken in adultery: "Let him among ye who is without sin cast the first stone." No wonder that the outcast woman kissed His feet and poured out the precious ointment upon Him. He was the Friend to such as she.

THE SEVENTH LESSON

THE BEGINNING OF THE END

The ministry of Jesus went on in about the same channels. Wandering here and there throughout the country, preaching and teaching in this town and that village, gathering around Him new followers, Jesus continued His work. He adapted Himself to His audience, giving to each what it needed, and not making the mistake of speaking over the heads of the people. He gave the general public the broad general teachings that they required, but He reserved the Inner Teachings for the Inner Circle of His followers whom He knew to be fit to receive the same. In this He showed a deep knowledge of men, and a strict accordance with the established custom of the mystics, who never make the mistake of giving the higher spiritual mathematics to the students who are learning the addition, subtraction and division rules of the occult. He cautioned His apostles regarding this point of teaching, even going so far as warning them positively and strongly against "casting pearls before swine."

One night He was in a boat crossing the lake of Gennesaret, in company with some of His fisherman followers. Tired out by the strenuous work of the day, He wrapped Himself up in His robe and fell into a deep sleep, from which He was later awakened by a noise and commotion among the crew and passengers. A terrible lake storm had sprung up, and the little vessel was tossing and pitching about among the waves in a manner which gave concern to even the experienced fishermen who manned her. The sails had been torn off, carrying away with them a portion of the mast, and the boat refused to respond to her rudder, the steering gear being rendered useless. The crew became panic-stricken and rushing to Jesus besought Him to save them from death in the storm. "Master! Master! Help ere we perish. The boat is foundering! Save us, Master!"

The Master arose and, using His occult power, caused the winds to cease their tempestuous activity, and the waves to become calm. He followed the Oriental occultists' custom of voicing His commands in words, not that the words had any virtue in themselves, but because they served a vehicle for His concentrated thought and focused will which He was using in his manifestation of occult power. With this knowledge of the process, occultists smile when they read the naïve account of the occurrence in the Gospels, where Jesus is described as addressing and rebuking the rebellious winds and then gently and kindly soothing the waters with words of "Peace, be still!" The fishermen who witnessed the occurrence, and from whom the reports thereof spread among the people, not understanding the nature of occult manifestations, thought that He was addressing the winds as actual entities, rebuking them and bidding them cease their vicious work, and soothing the sea in the same manner.

They did not comprehend the mental processes back of the words, and in their simplicity thought that He was actually rebuking the wind and soothing the waters. All occultists know that in "treating" material conditions the process is rendered much easier and simpler if we will but think of and "speak to" the condition as if it had intelligence and actual being, thus more easily directing the forces.

Obeying the thought and will of the Master, the winds abated their fury and the waters ceased their troubling. Gradually the boat rested easily upon the bosom of the lake, and the crew breathed freely once more, and then began their work of righting the mast and steering gear. And they wondered as they worked and asked each other "What manner of man is this, whom even the winds and the waters obey?" And Jesus, looking sadly at them, voiced that cry of the mystic who knows of the inherent and latent powers of man over material conditions, awaiting the exercise of the Will that may be exercised only in response to a great Faith. He answered them, saying, "Oh, ye of little Faith. What had you to fear?"

To the mystic it seems strange that people are able to read the Gospel accounts of the above and similar events and yet see no more in them than a mere recital of miracles wrought by some supernatural power. To the reader who has learned the fundamental truths, the New Testament record of the wonder-working of Jesus, even as imperfect as that record is, is full of advanced occult instructions stated so plainly that it seems as if even the casual reader must recognize it. But no, the old rule is still in force—each reads only that for which he is ready—each must bring something to a book, before he may expect to take anything away from it—to him that hath shall be given. Ever the same old mystic truth, manifest ever and ever, at all times and in all places. It is a fundamental law of the mind.

The journey across the lake was attended by another manifestation of occult power which is often passed over by the church teachers without comment, or at least with a labored endeavor to "explain" the evident meaning of the narrative. The modern materialistic trend of thought has invaded even the churches and has caused the preachers and teachers to endeavor to escape the accusation of "believing in spirits" and similar phenomena of the Astral World.

When the company reached the coast of Gergesa, on the opposite side of the lake, it disembarked and Jesus and His disciples pressed in toward the coast towns. As they passed among the cliffs lining the shore, they perceived two uncanny wandering figures which, gibbering, followed them along. The two maniacs, for such they were, approached the party, and one of them began to address the Master in a strange manner, beseeching Him to relieve the two of the devils possessing them. He called aloud, "O Master, thou Son of the Living God, have mercy upon us, and drive away the unclean things that we have allowed to enter into us."

The Gospels say nothing regarding the cause of this demoniac obsession, and the preachers prefer to pass over it rapidly, or else to treat it as a delusion of the insane, notwithstanding the direct statement of the New Testament narrative and its sequel or concluding statement. But the occult traditions have it that these two men were victims of their dabbling into certain phases of psychic phenomena, i.e., the "raising up of spirits" by the arts of Black Magic. In other words, these men had been experimenting along the lines of Jewish Necromancy, or Invocation and Evocation of Disembodied Astral Intelligences by means of Conjuration. They had raised up Astral Intelligences that had then refused to retire to their own plane, but which had taken possession of the physical organisms of their invokers and had remained in possession, causing the men to be regarded as maniacs, which resulted in their becoming outcasts among the caves with which the cliffs abounded, the same places being also the tombs of the dead. We do not wish to go into details here regarding this matter, but we wish to give the occult explanation of this little understood "miracle" of Jesus, which, however, is clearly understood by all occultists.

Jesus fully understood the nature of the trouble, and began at once to drive out these invading Astral Intelligences by means of his occult power. In a few moments, a cry was heard from the hills near by, and a great herd of swine were seen rushing down the hill, and in a moment were over the precipice and were soon drowned. The Gospel narrative is perfectly plain on this subject—it states that the legions of devils had passed from the men into the swine and the latter had plunged in terror into the water and were drowned. Jesus had distinctly and positively spoken to the demons, calling them "unclean spirits," and bidding them "come out" of the men. And all advanced students of Occultism understand why the pigs were used as intermediate instruments of the driving back of the Astral Intelligences to their own plane of life, which reason, however, is not in place or keeping in this work intended for general public reading.

The maniacs were restored to their normal condition, and the traditions say that the Master instructed them regarding the evil courses which they had been pursuing, and bade them desist from their nefarious practices which had wrought such evil consequences upon them.

The church and its preachers, with but few exceptions, have seen fit to ignore the frequent Biblical allusions to "devils," "demons," etc.; their position being practically that the writers of the events of Jesus' ministry (whom they otherwise consider to have been "inspired") must have been superstitious, credulous people believing in "the absurd demonology of their times." They ignore the fact that Jesus Himself repeatedly spoke to these intelligences, bidding them depart from the people whom they had been obsessing. Does the church wish to hold that the Master was also an ignorant, credulous peasant, sharing popular superstitions? It would seem so. We must except the Catholic Church from this criticism, for its authorities have recognized the true state of affairs and have warned its followers against indulging in the dark practices of Necromancy or Invocation of Astral Intelligences.

Occult science informs its students of the various planes of life, each of which contains its inhabitants. It teaches that on the Astral Plane there are disembodied entities which should not be transplanted to our plane. And it warns all against the dark practices, so common in ancient times and in the Middle Ages, of invoking and evoking these undesirable denizens of that plane. It is to be regretted that some of the modern Psychic Researchers ignore these plain warnings, for some of them are laying themselves open to grave consequences by reason of their wilful folly. We urge upon our readers to refrain from this dabbling in the phenomena of the Astral Plane. Some writer has well compared "Psychism" to a great machine, in the cog-wheels of which persons may become entangled only to be afterward drawn into the machine itself. Keep away from the wheels!

This "miracle" of Jesus aroused great excitement, and it was urged against Him that He was going about the country driving devils into people's flocks and herds, causing their destruction. The priests fomented the popular feeling, and encouraged the distrust, hatred and fear which the orthodox portion of the community was beginning to entertain toward the Master. The seeds of Calvary were being sown among the people. And their awful fruit was latent in them. Hate and bigotry were the essence of both seed and fruit.

Jesus returned to Capernaum, and once more the little town was crowded with people seeking instruction and crying to be healed. The news of his wonderful healing power spread far and near, and people were carried on litters for many miles in order that they might be touched by the hands of the Master.

About this time there came to Him one Jairus, a man of eminence in the community and in the church. Jairus had a little daughter about twelve years of age, who was taken seriously ill, and who had been given up as incurable by the physicians.

With his daughter lying at death's door, Jairus hastened to the scene of the Master's meetings, and, throwing himself at His feet, besought Him to heal his beloved child ere she passed beyond the dark portals of the unknown. The Master, feeling compassion for the father's great grief, paused in His teaching and started toward Jairus' home. His mind charged with the concentration of healing thought, and His organism filled with the vital forces aroused to perform the task, He felt some one touch the hem of His garment in search of healing power, and He at once recognized the occurrence, saying, "The power hath been drawn from me. Who touched my garment?" As they approached the house of Jairus, the servants came running out with wild cries and lamentations, announcing that the child had died while awaiting the coming of the Healer. The father broke down at this terrible news, coming at the very moment of his greatest hope. But Jesus bade him to have faith and still believe. Then, accompanied by three of His disciples—John, Peter and James—He entered the chamber of death. Waving back the weeping family and the neighbors who had gathered, "Stand back," He cried, "the child is not dead—she but sleepeth."

An indignant cry went up from the orthodox relatives and friends at these words of the Master. How dared He so mock the very presence of the dead, whom the physicians had left, and over whom the priests had already begun the last sacred rites? But, heeding them not, the Master passed His hands over the child's head, and took her little cold palms within his own. Then began a strange happening. The little chest began to heave, and the white wan cheeks began to show traces of color. Then the arms and hands began to move, and the wasted limbs drew slightly up. Then, opening her eyes with a wondering look, the child gazed at the Healer and smiled gently at Him. Then the Master, with a look of gentle tenderness, withdrew from the room, after ordering that nourishing food be brought for the child.

Then began the usual dispute. Some declared that another had been raised from the dead, while others declared that the child had but been in a trance and would have awakened anyway. Had not even the Healer declared that she only slept? But Jesus heeded not the disputants, but returned to the scene of His work.

The work went on in its accustomed way. He began to send His apostles away on longer and more extended tours, having fully instructed them in the occult methods of healing. Great success attended their efforts and the best reports came in from all sides. The authorities recognized to a still greater extent the growing influence of the young Master, and His actions were still more closely watched by the spies. Reports of His teachings and work were carried to Herod, who, recognizing in them the same note that had been struck by John the Baptist, who had been put to death, perceived that though men might die, the spirit of their teachings would still live on. No wonder the guilty ruler should cry in terror, "This verily is the spirit of John, whom I put to death, risen from the grave to wreak vengeance upon me!" And the authorities reported to Rome that here was a young fanatic, whom many believed to be the Messiah and coming King of the Jews, who had thousands of followers all over the land. And word came back from Rome, in due time, to watch carefully over the man, who was undoubtedly striving to incite an insurrection, and to imprison Him or put Him to death as soon as the evidence was sufficient to convict Him.

Jesus about this time was near a small fishing town called Bethseda, on the lake about seven miles from Capernaum. Near this place His boat landed at a place on the beach where He had hoped to take a few days' rest. But, alas, a great crowd had hastened to the place of disembarkation, and now gathered around Him, demanding teaching and healing. Putting aside His mental and physical fatigue, He attended to the wants of the crowd. Healing now, and then teaching, He threw Himself into His work with fervor and zeal. There were over five thousand people gathered together around Him, and toward evening the cry went up that there was not sufficient food in the camp to begin to feed the multitude. A great tumult arose among the crowd, and complaints and even curses began to be heard. The spiritual wants were forgotten, and the physical began to manifest itself in a most insistent manner. What was to be done?

He called together those of His company who had been entrusted with the care of the food which the little company carried with it. And, to His sorrow, He learned that the entire stock of food consisted of five loaves of bread and two fishes. And the little band carried practically no money with it, for they depended upon the hospitality of the country and the offerings by the faithful. The disciples advised that the Master order the crowd to disperse and return to Bethseda for food. But Jesus felt loath to do this, particularly when there were so many invalids in the gathering who had traveled so many miles to see Him, and who had not yet been healed. And so He decided to give the company its food by means of His power.

He bade His people divide the multitude into little groups of fifty people, who were then instructed to be seated for a meal. Then He ordered the scanty supply of available food to be brought before Him, and, placing His hands over it, He offered a blessing, then ordered His people to serve the throng. They began to serve out the food with looks of wonder and amazement. Had the Master lost His senses? But in some way the food seemed miraculously to increase and multiply, until at last all of the five thousand had been fully supplied and their hunger appeased. And then, after all had been served and had eaten, the scraps and fragments which were gathered up filled many wicker baskets and were distributed to the poorer people in the company for tomorrow's use.

But trouble arose. The people, with well filled stomachs, feeling that here indeed was royal bounty and the power with which to feed them forever free of charge, began to wax enthusiastic and shouts ascended. "The Messiah! King of the Jews! Provider of the People! Son of David! Ruler over Israel!" were the words which soon swept the crowd off of its feet. And then some of the bolder ones, or else the hired spies who wished to place Him in a compromising position, began to suggest that the crowd form itself into an army and march from city to city with Jesus at its head, until at last they would place Him upon the throne of Israel at Jerusalem. Jesus, recognizing the peril to His mission, managed to dissuade the hotheads from their plans, but still fearing that the authorities might come down upon the assemblage, ordered that the Twelve take the boat and put out for the other side of the lake. He sent them off as a precaution, but He, Himself, remained with the crowd and faced the threatened danger.

He retired to the hills near by and spent the night in meditation. Then early in the morning, He noticed that a storm was rising over the lake and that the tiny boat containing His disciples would be in great danger. In a few moments they might be overwhelmed. He wished to be with them to comfort and re-assure them. No boat being handy, he stepped boldly out upon the water and walked rapidly toward the direction in which He knew the boat must be. Scarcely conscious of the occult power of levitation that He was using to overcome the power of gravitation, He moved rapidly toward His followers. Soon He overtook them, and they, seeing a white figure moving swiftly over the water toward them, were affrighted, believing it to be a spirit or ghost. "It is I, be not afraid!" called out the Master to them. Then Peter cried out, "Lord, if Thou it be, direct me to walk to Thee also on the waves!" And the Master, smiling, so directed him. And Peter, whose latent occult power was aroused by his great faith in the Master, sprang over the side and took several steps toward Him. But, suddenly losing his faith and courage, his power also left him, and he began to sink beneath the waves. But the Master grasped his hand and led him in safety to the boat and both entered it. Then the crew fell to and with great enthusiasm righted the boat and proceeded to the shore near Capernaum.

In the case of Peter and his experience in walking on the water, we have a striking instance of the well known power of the mental attitude of Faith in the manifestation of occult power. All occultists know this, and without feeling an implicit faith in the Power with them, they do not attempt certain forms of manifestation. They know that with Faith miracles may be performed which are impossible otherwise. So long as Peter held his Faith he was able to counteract certain laws of nature by means of other laws not so well known. But as soon as Fear took the place of Faith his power left him. This is an invariable occult principle, and in the recital of this story of Peter on the water is to be found a whole volume of occult instruction—to those who are able to read it.

Arriving safely on the shores of the lake, Jesus resumed His work while the ever-present gathering of people went on in its accustomed way. But on the opposite shore of the lake the crowd who had been fed on the loaves and fishes were in an angry mood. They cried out that they had been deserted by their leader, and that the expected loaves and fishes—the free meals that they had expected would continue—had been denied them. They also complained bitterly that the reign of miracles had not continued. And they began to revile the Master that they had acclaimed the night before. And so Jesus experienced the ingratitude and the unreasonable words of the public just as all great teachers have done. The seekers after the loaves and the fishes, demanding to be fed and clothed without their own work—the seekers after miracles, demanding fresh wonder-workings—have ever been the bane of the great Teachers of the Truth. It is a hard and bitter truth, but all teachers and true lovers of the Truth must learn to meet and understand it. The mob which reveres a spiritual Master today is equally ready to rend him to pieces tomorrow.

And still more trouble arose from this mistaken kindness which led Jesus to feed the crowd by His occult powers, which, by the way, He knew to be in opposition to the well-established custom of the Occult Brotherhoods. The formalists, Pharisees and Scribes, having heard of the occurrence, gathered about the Master and accused Him of violating one of the forms and ceremonies prescribed by the ecclesiastical authorities—the rite which required the faithful to wash their hands before beginning a meal. They accused Him of heresy and false teaching, which tended to lead the people away from their accustomed ceremonies and observances. Jesus waxed indignant and, turning on His critics, hurled burning replies upon them. "Ye hypocrites!" He cried, "You cling to the commandments of men and neglect the commandments of God! You cleanse your hands but not your souls! You are the blind leaders of the blind, and both yourselves and your followers fall in the mire and ditches! Away with you and your hypocrisy!" But the adverse comment aroused by His actions would not down, and, discouraged and disheartened by the evidences of the barrenness of the soil in which He had been sowing the precious seeds of the Truth, He gathered together His followers and departed into Tyre and Sidon, a quieter region, that He might rest and meditate over new plans and work. He could see the beginning of the end.

To understand the nature of the position of the Master at this time, it must be remembered that His strong hold had ever been with the masses of the people, who were His enthusiastic admirers. So long as He remained entrenched in the heart of the populace, the temporal and ecclesiastical authorities dared not attack Him without a popular uprising of no mean proportions. But now that they had managed to wean away His public from Him they pressed Him harder and harder with their persecutions and complaints. And so at last they had managed to render Him almost an unpopular outcast. They forced Him away from the larger towns, and now He was wandering among the less populous regions of the country, and even there the spies and agents of the authorities hunted Him down, seeking to further entrap and compromise Him.

About this time Jesus revealed to His apostles the facts of His Divine origin which was now plain to Him. He also told them of the fate which awaited Him, and which He had willingly chosen. He told them not to expect the fruits of His work at this time, for He was but sowing the seeds of the fruit which would not grow and bear fruit for many centuries. He gave them the Mystic secret of the nature of

His work, which is taught to the Initiates of the Occult Brotherhoods even unto this day. But even these chosen men scarcely grasped the true import of His teachings, and once He was rendered almost broken hearted at over-hearing a discussion among them regarding high offices which they hoped to acquire.

Jesus now felt that the time had come for Him to move on to Jerusalem to meet there the crowning act of His strange career. And, knowing full well that such a course would be virtually thrusting His head into the very jaws of the lion of ecclesiastical and temporal authority, He set His feet firmly on the road which led to Jerusalem, the capital city, and the center of ecclesiastical influence. And that road was a hard one to travel, for, as He neared the capital, His enemies increased in number and the opposition to Him grew stronger. At one village He had been denied the right of shelter, an indignity almost unknown in Oriental lands. In another place a large rock was hurled at Him and wounded Him severely. The mob had turned against Him and was repaying His kind services with abuse and personal violence. And this is ever the lot of the teacher of the Truth who scatters the sacred pearls of Truth before the swine of the unworthy multitude of people. Over and over again has this fact been brought home to those who would labor for the good of the world. And still we hear the querulous complaint that the Inner Teaching is reserved for the Few—why not scatter it broadcast among the people? The stake, the rack, the stones, the prison cell, the cross and their modern prototypes—these are the silent answers to the question.

Moving on toward Jerusalem the little company reached Perea, a number of miles from Bethany, at which latter place dwelt a family of His friends—the two sisters, Martha and Mary, and their brother Lazarus. At this place He was met by a messenger from Bethany, who bore the sad news that His friend Lazarus was sick unto death, and who also begged the Master to return to Bethany and cure the man. But this Jesus refused to do, and allowed several days to pass without answering the summons. At the end of the several days He started toward Bethany, telling His disciples that Lazarus was dead. And reaching Bethany they found that it was indeed so—Lazarus was dead and in the tomb.

Jesus was received with scowling antagonism. The people seemed to say, "Here is this heretical imposter again. He feared to come even to the aid of His dying friend. His power has failed Him and He now stands discredited and exposed!" Then came Martha, who reproached the Master with His indifference and delay. He answered her that Lazarus should rise again, but she doubted His word. Then came Mary, whose grief brought tears even from the Master, who had seen so much of human suffering as to have found his eyes refuse to weep.

Then asked the Master, "Where have you laid him away?" and they took Him to the tomb, followed by the curious mob hungering for the sight of more wonders from the man whom they feared even while hating and reviling Him. Jesus stood before the dreary tomb and bade the men roll away the stone that closed the mouth of the tomb. The men hesitated, for they knew that a corpse lay within, and they even perceived the characteristic odor of the tomb issuing therefrom. But the Master insisting upon it, they rolled away the stone and Jesus stood full in front of the dark opening to the cavern.

He stood there for a few moments wrapt in meditation and showing evidences of strong mental concentration. His eyes took on a strange look, and in every muscle He showed that He was summoning to the task every particle of the power at His command. He was throwing off the matters that had been occupying His mind during the past weeks, that He might hold his mind "one-pointed," as the Oriental occultists term it—that He might concentrate clearly and forcibly upon the task before Him.

Then, arousing His reserve force, in a mighty effort, He cried loudly, in a voice of authority and power, "Lazarus! Lazarus! Come forth!"

The people gasped with horror at this calling forth a corpse which was in the process of disintegration and decay, and a cry of remonstrance went up, but Jesus heeded it not. "Lazarus! Lazarus! Come forth, I command thee!" he cried again.

And then at the mouth of the cavern could be seen something startling. It was a ghastly figure, bound and clad in the grave-clothes of that country, which was struggling to free itself and to move toward the light. It was indeed Lazarus! And, after tearing off the stained grave-clothes which still retained the horrid stench of decaying matter, his body was found to be sweet and clean and pure as that of the infant. Jesus had performed a wonder-work far beyond any manifestation He had heretofore shown to the world.

The excitement occasioned by this crowning wonder, coming to Jerusalem after a lull in which it had thought that the Master had retired into insignificant seclusion, aroused again into activity the authorities, who now determined to make an end to the matter and to suppress this pestilent charlatan once and for all. Raising a decaying corpse from the tomb, indeed! What new fraudulent marvels would He not work next in order to delude the credulous people and to bring them once more around his rebellious standard? The man was dangerous without doubt, and must be put where He could do no harm—and that at once.

Within a few hours after the receipt of news that Lazarus had walked from the tomb, the Sanhedrin, the great Jewish ecclesiastical council, was in session, called hastily by its officers to take vigorous action concerning this impious, heretical imposter who had been allowed to mock at established order and religion for too long a time. He must be quieted ere he arouse the people once more. The Roman authorities were warned by the Jewish ecclesiastics that this dangerous man now approaching the capital claimed to be the Jewish Messiah, and that His aims were to overturn the Temple authorities first, and then establish Himself as King of the Jews, and place Himself at the head of a revolutionary army which would attempt to defy and defeat the rule of mighty Rome herself.

And so all the machinery was set in motion, and the officers of the law were all on the alert to take advantage of the first overt act of Jesus and His followers, and to throw them into prison as enemies of society, religion and of the state. The Roman authorities were agitated at the reports coming to them from the highest Jewish authorities, and were prepared to crush the rebellion at the first sign. The Jewish priests were in solemn convocation and at the instigation of Caiaphas, the high priest of the Jews, they determined that nothing but the death of this false Messiah would put an end to the agitation which threatened to drive them from power and authority. And so the die was cast.

And meanwhile Jesus was resting in Bethany, surrounded by great throngs who were pouring into the place to see Lazarus, and to renew their allegiance to the Master whom they had so basely forsaken. Time-servers ever, the latest miracles had revived their fading interest and waning faith, and they flocked around the Master as noisy, enthusiastic and as full of fulsome praise as ever. And yesterday they had damned Him, and tomorrow they would cry "Crucify Him!" For such is the nature of the multitude of men. Of the multitudes of Jesus' followers, none remained to acknowledge allegiance in His hour of arrest—even among the chosen twelve, one betrayed Him, one denied Him, and all fled away when He was taken captive. And for such the Son of Man lived and taught and suffered. Surely His life was the greatest miracle of all.

THE EIGHTH LESSON

THE END OF THE LIFE WORK

Resting for a short time before His formal entry into Jerusalem, the Master sought the seclusion of the sparsely settled districts near the wilderness. In and around the village of Ephraim, in Perea, in parts of Galilee, He wandered with the Twelve. But even there He continued His work of healing and teaching.

But even this temporary respite from the inevitable lasted but a short time. Jesus determined to march direct to the seat of the ecclesiastical and temporal authority which was arrayed against Him. And so, just before the coming of the Passover time, He gathered together the Twelve and set out on the final stage of the journey. The pilgrims journeying to the capital were burning with curiosity and excitement concerning this journey of the Master to the home of His foes. Rumors were circulated that He intended to gather His forces together and sweep the enemy from its seats of power. It was known that the Sanhedrin intended to attempt to punish Him, and the people asked why should He move on to face His foes unless He contemplated a fight to the finish?

This belief in His determination caused a revulsion of feeling of the people in His favor, and many who had deserted Him now again gathered around Him. They dreamt again of victory, and scented again an unfailing supply of loaves and fishes. They crowded around Him wishing to be among the victorious host. But He encouraged them not—neither spoke He a word to them. He knew them for the time-servers that they were.

The crowds of Jerusalem hearing of His approach, and moved by curiosity to witness His triumphant entry into the City, flocked around the suburbs through which He would approach. At last the cry went up, "Here He comes!" and to their amazement and disgust the crowd saw Him riding quietly info the City mounted on an ass, without display, pretense or pose. The crowd scattered, sneering and reviling Him. But the pilgrims were becoming more and more enthusiastic, and they strewed His way with palms, shouting, "Blessed be our Messiah! The King of Israel approacheth."

The Master proceeded directly to the Temple and performed the customary rites. So amazed were the authorities by His fearless demeanor, that they deferred laying violent hands upon Him. They feared a trap, and moved cautiously. They even allowed Him to retire to Bethany and spend the night. The next morning He returned to the city and dwelt among His friends there. He attended the Temple regularly, and pursued His work of teaching and healing in its very shadows.

Meanwhile the clouds of the persecuting forces gathered closely around His head. One of the Twelve, Judas Iscariot, who was sorely disappointed at the Master having refused to take advantage of the support of the crowd to assist His claim as the Messiah and King of the Jews, and also fearing that he would become involved in His inevitable downfall, began a series of bargainings and dickerings with the authorities, which had for their object the betrayal of the Master into the hands of the authorities, the reward to be immunity from persecution for himself and a few pieces of silver for his pocket in addition.

And so the time passed on, the nights being spent at Bethany and the days at the Temple in the capital. Finally the priests made an important move. They confronted Him in their official capacity and demanded that He prove His ordination as a Jewish Rabbi and consequent right to preach to the orthodox members of the church. Jesus answered them by asking questions that they feared to answer. Then they began to question Him, hoping to involve Him in ecclesiastical heresies which would give them their excuse to arrest Him. But He evaded them skilfully. They sought also to compel Him to state opinions contrary to the Roman authority, but He likewise escaped this net.

Finally, however, they drew from Him a savage attack upon authority, and He cried out in indignation:

"Woe unto you, ye generation of vipers! Ye serpents! Ye hypocrites! Ye oppressors of the poor! Ye professed shepherds, who are but as wolves in disguise, seeking but to devour the sheep whom ye have in charge! Woe unto you, ye Scribes, Hypocrites, Pharisees!"

Then He left the Temple and returned to Bethany to spend the night, after foretelling the destruction of the Temple, when there should not be left one of its stones upon another.

That night he had a heart-to-heart talk with the Twelve. He told them that the end was in sight—that He was to die before many hours had passed—that they, the Twelve, were to become wanderers on the face of the earth—hunted and persecuted in His name and for His sake. A terrible revelation to some among them who had dreamt of earthly grandeur and high positions for themselves! And then Judas felt that the time to act had come, and he stole away to meet the High-priest and to close the frightful bargain with him which was to make his name the synonym for treachery throughout the ages.

The next day, Wednesday, He rested in Bethany the whole twenty-four hours, evidently gathering together his reserve forces to meet the ordeal which He now knew was before Him. He kept apart from even His disciples and spent the time in meditation. And likewise was passed the early part of the following day, Thursday. But when the even time had come, He sent for the Twelve and gathered them around Him for the Paschal Supper, one of the rites of the Passover time.

Even this last solemn occasion was marred by a petty squabble among the disciples regarding the order of precedence to be observed in their seats at the table. Judas succeeded in gaining the seat of honor next to the Master. Jesus startled the company by insisting upon washing the feet of the Twelve, an act which placed them on a pedestal above Him. This occult ceremony, which was not comprehended by the Twelve, apparently was one which the Hierophants of the Occult Brotherhoods performed for their associates when the latter had been chosen to carry out some important office or mission, or when a successor was about to take the place of one of them. And Jesus evidently so intended it. Then He bade them wash one another's feet, in token of the recognition of each of the high mission of the others.

Then Jesus, overcome by the knowledge of the morrow, burst out in anguished tones, saying: "And even one of you, my chosen ones, shall betray me!" And several asked Him in turn, in a tone of reproach, "Is it I?" And Jesus shook His head at each question. But Judas asked not, but overcome with confusion he reached over and took a portion of bread from the plate before the Master. Then Jesus took a bit of bread and, moistening it from His plate, handed it to Judas, saying to him firmly, "Judas, do thy work without loss of time." And Judas, abashed, slunk away from the table.

Then began that remarkable conversation of the Last Supper, as recorded in the Gospels. Then also was performed that first celebration of the Holy Communion, the Mystic significance of which shall be explained in a later lesson. Then Jesus chanted the Passover hymn.

Then shortly after, the company left the room and walked into the streets, and over the meadows near by. Then under the trees of the Garden of Gethsemane, apart from His disciples, now reduced to Eleven, He gave Himself up to prayer and meditation. He called aloud to The Father to give Him strength for the final ordeal. Struggling with His doubts and fears and misgivings—conquering His physical inclination and impulses—He gave utterance to that supreme cry: "O Father, Thy will, not mine, be done!" and in so saying He cast behind Him forever His right of choice to stay the awful course of events which was pressing upon Him. Resigning His mighty occult power of defense, He laid Himself upon the altar of sacrifice even as the Paschal Lamb.

Leaving behind Him the Garden in which He had just performed this greatest miracle of all—the miracle of Renunciation—He stepped out among His disciples, saying, "The hour has come—the betrayer is here to do his work."

Then were heard sounds of clanking arms, and martial tread, and in a moment the military guard appeared on the scene, accompanied by a delegation of ecclesiastics, and with them, walking in advance, was Judas Iscariot. Judas, walking as one in a trance, approached the Master and, saluting Him with a kiss, cried, "Hail, Master," which was the signal to the guard, arranged between Judas and the High Priest. Then cried Jesus, "Ah, with a kiss—thou, Judas, betrayeth the Son of Man with a kiss! Oh!" And in that moment it seemed that the Master's grief had reached its utmost limit. Then the guard closed around Him and carried Him away.

But He resisted them not. As they approached Him He called out, "Whom seek ye?" And the leader answered, "We seek him whom men call Jesus of Nazareth." Then answered the Master, "I am He whom thou seeketh!" But the disciples resisted the arrest, and Peter cut off the ear of one of the party, a servant of the Highpriest. But Jesus bade His followers desist, and, approaching the wounded man, placed his severed ear in place and healed it instantly. Then He rebuked His disciples, telling them that, had He so desired, the whole of the legions of heaven would have come to His assistance. Then He bade the leader conduct Him from the place. But alas! as He left, He turned to bid farewell to His disciples, and lo! to a man they had fled and deserted Him, leaving Him alone in His hour of trial—yea! as every humble soul must be alone in its moments of supreme struggle—alone with its Creator.

Then down toward the city they led Him—the Master of All Power, an humble captive, non-resistant and awaiting the course of The Will. They took Him to the palace of the Jewish High-priest, where the Sanhedrin was assembled in secret session awaiting His coming. And there He stood erect before these ecclesiastical tyrants to be judged—bound with the cord as a common criminal. He, whose single effort of His will would have shattered the whole palace to pieces and have destroyed every human being within its walls!

And this was but the beginning. During the next eight hours He was subjected to six separate trials, if indeed such mock proceedings might be so designated. Subjected to blows, and all manner of low insults, the Master remained a Master. Perjured witnesses testified, and all manner of crimes and heresies were charged against Him. Then Caiaphas asked Him the all-important question, "Art thou the Christ?" and Jesus broke His silence to answer positively, "I am!" Then the High-priest cried out vehemently, rending His sacred robes in his pious indignation, "He has blasphemed!"

From that moment there was no possible chance of escape for the Master. He had virtually condemned Himself by His own words. There was no retreat or reprieve. He was roughly pushed from the hall and like a common criminal was turned over to the taunts and revilings of the mob, which availed itself of its privileges to the full in this case. Insults, curses, revilings, taunts, and even blows, came fast and furiously upon Him. But He stood it all without a murmur. Already His thoughts had left earthly things behind, and dwelt on planes of being far above the wildest dreams of men. With His mind firmly fixed on the Real, the Unreal vanished from His consciousness.

In the early part of the day following the night of His arrest, Jesus was taken before Pontius Pilate, the Roman official, for His trial by the civil authorities. Pilate, in his heart, was not disposed to condemn Jesus, for he believed that the whole trouble consisted in theological and ecclesiastical differences with which the civil law should not concern itself. His wife had warned him against becoming involved in the dispute, for she had a secret sympathy for the Master, for some reason. But he found arrayed against him the solid influence of the Jewish priesthood, whose power must not be opposed lightly, according to the policy of Rome. Then the priests had made out a civil case against Jesus, claiming that He had sought to incite a rebellion and proclaim Himself King of the Jews; that He had created public disorder; that He had urged the people to refuse to pay taxes to Rome. The case against Him was weak, and Pilate was at a loss what to do. Then some one of the priests suggested that as Jesus was a Galilean, He be turned over for trial to Herod, in whose territory the principal crimes were committed, and Pilate gladly availed himself of this technical excuse to rid himself of responsibility in the matter. And so the case was transferred to Herod, who happened to be in Jerusalem at that time on a visit. To

Herod's palace the captive was taken, and after suffering indignities and humiliation at the hand of the tyrant, He was remanded back to Pilate for trial, under Herod's orders.

Back to Pilate's court, followed by the crowd, went Jesus. Pilate was greatly annoyed that Herod should have shifted the responsibility once more upon his (Pilate's) court. Then he bethought himself of an expedient. He took advantage of the Jewish custom, observed by the Roman rulers, which led to the pardoning of a notorious criminal on the occasion of the Passover. And so he announced that he would pardon Jesus according to custom. But from the Jewish authorities came back the answer that they would not accept Jesus as the subject of the pardon, but demanded that Barabbas, a celebrated criminal, be pardoned instead of the Nazarene. Pilate found himself unable to escape the designs of the Jewish priesthood, and so, yielding in disgust, he pardoned Barabbas, and condemned Jesus to death. The cries of the mob, incited by the priests, sounded around the court. "Crucify him! Crucify him!" Pilate appeared before the priests and the populace, and, washing his hands in a basin, according to the Oriental custom, he cried to the Jews, "I wash my hands of this man's blood—upon you be it!" And the crowd responded with a great shout, "Upon us and our children be his blood!"

Jesus, in the meantime, had been cruelly scourged by the barbarous instruments of torture of the time. His body was lacerated and bleeding, and He was faint from the torture and loss of blood. Upon His head had been thrust, in ghastly mockery, a crown of thorns which pressed deep into His flesh. He was refused the usual respite of several days before sentence and execution—He was to die that very day.

His cross was tied to His back and He was compelled to carry it, fainting though He was from fatigue and torture. He staggered along and fell, unable to bear His heavy burden. Finally Golgotha, the place of the crucifixion, was reached, and the Man of Sorrows was nailed to the cross and raised aloft to die a lingering and painful death. On either side was a criminal—two thieves—His companions in suffering.

He refused to partake of the drug which was granted to criminals to relieve their intense suffering. He preferred to die in full possession of His faculties. Above His head was a tablet bearing the inscription, "The King of the Jews," which had been placed there by Pilate in a spirit of ironical mockery of the Jews who had forced him to place this man on the cross.

As the cross was raised into position the Master cried aloud, "O Father, forgive them—they know not what they do."

Taunted by the crowds, He hung and suffered the terrible agonies of the cross. Even one of the crucified criminals reviled Him, asking Him why He did not save Himself and them? The crowd asked Him why He who saved others could not save Himself? But He, who could have brought forces to bear which would have wrought the miracle they demanded, answered not, but awaited the end.

Then set in the delirium of death in which He cried aloud to the Father, asking if He had been forsaken in His misery. But the end was near.

There arose a strange storm—darkness fell over the place—weird electrical disturbances manifested themselves. The winds abated and a strange quiet fell over all the scene, which was lighted by a ghastly glow. And then came the earthquake, with strange groanings and moanings of the earth; with frightful stenches of sulphur and gas. And the very foundations of Jerusalem quaked and shivered. The rocks before the tombs flew off, and the dead bodies were exposed to view. In the Temple, the veil before the Holy of Holies was rent in twain.

The cries of the people as they rushed to and fro in mortal terror took the attention of all from the cross. Then the Roman officer in charge of the execution, glancing upward, saw that all was over, and, falling before the cross, he cried out, "Verily, this man was a god!"

Jesus the Master had passed out from the body which had served as His tenement for thirty-three years. His body was borne away for burial, in a secret place. Embalmed by loving friends, it was carried to a place of last earthly rest.

* * * * *

And now we come to a portion of the narrative in which the occult traditions and teachings diverge from the account stated in the Gospels. We should have said apparently diverge, for the two accounts vary only because of the varying points of view and different degrees of understanding of the teachers.

We allude to the events of the Resurrection.

It must be remembered that Jesus had informed His disciples that in three days He would "rise from the dead" and appear once more among them. To the ordinary understanding these events seem to indicate that the Master would once more occupy His physical body, and that His reappearance was to be so understood. And the Gospel narrative certainly seems to verify this idea, and was undoubtedly so stated that it might be more readily understood by the popular mind.

But the occult traditions hold otherwise. They hold that Jesus really appeared to His disciples three days after His death, and abode with them for a time teaching and instructing them in the deeper mysteries and secret doctrines. But the mystics have always held and taught that His reappearance was in the Astral Body, and not in the discarded physical form.

To the popular mind the physical body was almost everything, as we have shown in one of the earlier lessons of this series. So much was this so that the mass of the people expected that all mankind would arise from the dead at the Last Day clad in their former physical forms. And so, any other teaching would have been unintelligible to them.

But to the occultists and mystics who understood the truth about the more ethereal vehicles of the soul, such an idea appeared crude and unscientific, and they readily grasped the Inner Teachings regarding the Resurrection, and understood the reason why Jesus would use the Astral Body as the vehicle of His reappearance.

The Gospel narrative informs us that a guard was placed around the tomb to prevent the body being stolen and a consequent assertion of the Resurrection which the priests well knew to be expected. It further states that the tomb was sealed and guarded by a squad of Roman soldiers, but that notwithstanding these precautions the body of the Master actually came to life and emerged from the tomb, and that His followers were disturbed by the evidences that His body had been stolen.

The occult traditions, however, state that the close friends of Jesus, aided by a prominent Jew who was a secret believer, obtained from the willing Pilate a secret order which enabled them to deposit the body in a safe and secret resting place where it gradually resolved itself into the dust to which all that is mortal must return. These men knew that the Resurrection of the Master had naught to do with mortal fleshly form or body. They knew that the immaterial soul of the Master still lived and would reappear to them clad in the more ethereal body made manifest to their mortal senses. Every occultist will understand this without further comment. To others we advise that they read the occult teachings concerning the Astral Body and its characteristics. This is no place in which to again describe at length the phenomena of the Astral Body of Man.

* * * * *

The first to see the Master in His Astral Form was Mary of Magdala, a woman admirer and follower of her Lord. She was weeping beside the empty tomb, when looking up she saw a form approaching. The Astral Form was indistinct and unfamiliar, and at first she did not recognize it. Then a voice called her name, and looking up she saw the form growing more distinct and familiar, and she recognized the features of her Master.

* * * * *

More than this, the occult legends assert the truth of some of the traditions of the early Christian Church, namely, that in the three days succeeding the scene of Calvary there appeared in and around Jerusalem the disembodied forms of many persons who had died a short time previously. It is said that the Astral Bodies of many dead Jews revisited the scenes of their former life, and were witnessed by friends and relatives.

* * * * *

Then Jesus appeared in His Astral Body to the disciples. The traditions have it that two of the eleven met Him on the afternoon of the day when He first appeared to Mary—Easter Sunday. Strange to say, they did not at first recognize Him, although they walked the road with Him and afterward ate at the same table. This failure to recognize the Master is wholly beyond ordinary explanation and the churches make no real attempt to make it understandable. But the occult traditions say that Jesus had not wholly materialized His Astral Body at first, for reason of prudence, and that consequently His features were not distinctly and clearly marked; then at the meal He caused His features to be fully materialized so that the disciples might readily recognize Him. All occultists who have witnessed the materialization of an Astral Body will readily understand this statement. The orthodox theory of Jesus having reappeared in His physical body wholly fails to explain this nonrecognition by His disciples, who had been His everyday companions before His death. The slightest consideration should show which statement is nearer the bounds of reasonable probability.

Jesus remained visible to the chosen few for forty days. The testimony of several hundred people attested the fact. There are a number of mystic legends about some of His appearances, which are not mentioned in the Gospel narratives. One of these states that

He appeared before Pontius Pilate and forgave him for the part he had played in the tragedy. Another that Herod witnessed His form in his bedchamber. Another that He confronted the High-priests in the Temple and brought them to their knees in terror. Another that He came one night to the Eleven, who sat behind bolted doors in hiding, and saying to them, "Peace be unto you, my beloved," vanished from sight.

The Gospels record another appearance before the Eleven, upon which occasion Thomas, the doubter, satisfied himself of the identity of the Astral Body by placing his fingers in the wounds, which, of course, were reproduced in the Astral Form according to the well known laws regarding the same.

This coming and going of Jesus—these sudden appearances and disappearances—these manifestations of His form only to those whom He wished to see Him, and His concealment from those whom He desired to remain in ignorance of His return, all show conclusively to every occultist the nature of the vehicle which He used for manifestation upon His return. It would seem incredible that there could be any general doubt on the subject were the public informed on the laws concerning the Astral World phenomena.

* * * * *

The Gospel narrative shows that the disciples recognized that Jesus was not a "spirit" in the sense of being an airy, unsubstantial form. They felt His body, and saw Him eat—but what of that? The laws of materialization of Astral forms make it possible, under certain conditions, that the Astral Form become so thoroughly materialized that it may not only be seen but actually felt. Even the records of the English Society for Psychical Research prove this fact, leaving out of account the phenomena with which all advanced occultists are familiar.

Then, one day He appeared to the disciples, and they accompanied Him to the hills, Jesus talking to them regarding their future work on earth. He then bade them farewell, and began to fade away from their sight. The common account pictures Him as ascending into the air until out of sight, but the mystic account informs us that His astral form began to slowly dematerialize and He gradually faded away from the sight of His beloved followers, who stood gazing in wistful longing at His form which, each moment, grew more and more ethereal in structure, until finally the dematerialization was complete and His soul had cast off all material form, shape and substance, and so passed on to the higher planes of being.

* * * * *

In view of this explanation, does not the commonly accepted version seem childish and crude? Can any one at all familiar with the laws and phenomena of the land Behind the Veil, suppose that a physical body could or would pass on to the planes in which the ordinary forms of matter do not exist? Such ideas are fit only for minds which find it necessary to think of the "resurrection of the body" of all departed souls, in order to conceive of Immortality. To the occultist, the physical body is merely a temporary vehicle for the soul which the latter discards at the proper time. It has nothing to do with the real being of the soul. It is merely the shell which is discarded by the soul, as the chrysalis shell is discarded by the butterfly when it spreads its wings for its aerial flight into a new world.

All these ideas about the immortality of the mortal body are the product of materialistic minds unused to thinking of the higher planes of life, and unable to grasp even the mental concept regarding the same. Of the earth, earthly, are these conceptions and ideas. And the sooner that Christianity sheds them as discarded shells the sooner will the church experience that revival of true spirituality that devout souls see the need of, and for which they are so earnestly praying.

The churches are so wedded to materialistic thought that a preacher does not even hint at the existence of phases of life above the physical lest he be termed "a spiritualist" or accused of being "spooky." In the name of Truth, is the teaching, that man is a spiritual being, inconsistent with the teachings of Christ and the records of the Scripture? Must one forego all such beliefs, in favor of a heathenish creed of "physical body" resurrection of the dead—an immortality in the worn-out mortal body long since discarded? Which is the true spiritual teaching? Can there be any doubt regarding the same in a mind willing to think for itself? It seems sad that the orthodox churches do not see this, and cease forcing out of their congregations all thinkers who dare assert the existence of a soul independent of the physical body.

What is the use of a soul, if the physical bodies of the dead are to be resurrected in order that their owners may enjoy immortality? And where are the souls of these dead bodies now residing and abiding pending the coming of the Last Day? Are the souls of the dead with their bodies? If not, then they must be living a life independent of the physical body—and if such be the case, why should they afterward be required to take on their worn-out physical bodies which they have managed so well without during their disembodied life? What becomes of those who had diseased, deformed or frail bodies during their mortal life—will they be compelled to inhabit these bodies through all eternity? Will the owners of aged, worn out bodies be compelled to re-assume them at the Last Day? If not, why the necessity of a physical body at all, in the future life? Do the angels have physical bodies? If not, why should souls require them on higher planes? Think over these questions and then realize how materialistic is the current Christian conception, when compared with that of Mystic Christianity, which teaches spiritual evolution from lower to higher planes of being, and on to planes of being beyond even the faintest conception of men of the present day.

* * * * *

The occult traditions teach that during the forty days of Jesus' appearance in the Astral Body, He imparted many of the Higher Truths to His disciples. They state that He even took some of them out of their bodies and showed them the higher Astral Planes of Being. He also informed them regarding the real nature of His mission which He now clearly saw with His spiritual mind, the cloud of His mortal mind being now removed.

He told them that the real work of His followers was the sowing of the seed of the Truth, without regard to immediate results. He told them that the real fruition would not come for many centuries—yea, not until the passing of over two thousand years or more. He told them that the passage of the centuries would be like the preparing of the soil for the great work of the Truth, and that afar in the distance would be the real fruit season.

He taught them regarding the Second Coming of Christ, when the real Truth of His teachings should become apparent to mankind and the true Life of the Spirit should be lived by the race. He taught them that their work was to keep alight the Flame of the Spirit and to pass it on to worthy followers.

This and many other things He told them, before He passed on.

And the mystics teach that He still lives in the world, diffused among all the living souls on earth, striving ever to lead them to a recognition of the Real Self—the Spirit Within. He is with us ever as an Abiding Spirit, a Comforter, a Helper, an Elder Brother.

He is not gone from us! He is here with us now and forever, in Actual Spirit Communion!

The Lord hath indeed Risen—Risen from Mortal Form to Immortal Spiritual Existence!

THE NINTH LESSON

THE INNER TEACHINGS

The first and main phase of the Inner Teachings of Mystic Christianity is that connected with the Mystery of the Life of Jesus. The outer teachings give but an imperfect view of the real life and nature of the Master, and theologians have built up an edifice of dogmatic theory around the same. The Mystery of the Life of Jesus forms the subject of some important Inner Teachings of the Mystic Fraternities and Occult Brotherhoods, and is considered by them to be the foundation of the other teachings. And so we shall consider this phase of the subject at this point.

In the first place we must remember that the soul of Jesus was different from the souls of other men. His was a "virgin birth"—not in the commonly accepted sense of the term, but in the occult sense as explained in the second lesson of this series. His soul was fresh from the hand of the Creator—His spirit had not been compelled to work through repeated incarnations, pressing forward for expression through humble and ignoble forms. It was free from taint, and as pure as the Fountain from which is flowed. It was a virgin soul in every sense of the term.

This being so, it follows that it was not bound by the Karma of previous incarnations—as is the case with the ordinary soul. It had no entangling ties—it had no seeds of desire and action planted in previous lives, which were pressing forward toward expression in His life. He was a Free Spirit—an Unbound Soul. And therefore He was not only unbound by any Karma of His own, but was also free (by nature) from the Karma of the race or of the world.

The absence of personal Karma left Him free from the selfish personal Desire which binds men to the wheel of action and personal ambition. He had no desire or thought for personal aggrandizement or glory, and was perfectly free (by nature) to work for the good of the race as an outside observer and helper, without suffering the pains and sorrows of race-life, had He so wished. But He chose otherwise, as we shall see in a moment.

The absence of Race-Karma, or World-Karma, freed Him from the necessity of the pains of humanity, which are a part of its collective Karma. He would have been perfectly able to live a life absolutely free from the pains, trials and troubles that are the common lot of Man, owing to the Race-Karma. He would have escaped persecution, physical and mental pains, and even death, had He so elected. But He chose these things of His own free will, in order to accomplish the great work that He saw before Him as a World-Savior.

In order for Jesus to enact His part as the Redeemer and Savior of the race, it was necessary for Him to take upon Himself His share of the Karma of the race—virtually taking upon Himself the "sins of the world." Before He could lift the burden from the race of men, He must become a man among men.

To understand this more clearly we must remember that to a being such as Jesus—a soul free from Karma—there would be no such thing as temptation, longings, desires, or any of the mental states of the ordinary man with the Karma of successive past incarnations resting within him as seeds of action pressing forward ever for unfoldment and expression.

Jesus, the free soul, would have been practically an outside observer of the world's affairs, and not influenced by any of its ordinary incentives to action. In this state He could have aided the world as a teacher and instructor, but He would not have been able to accomplish His great task of Redeeming the world, in its highest spiritual significance, as we shall see as we proceed. It was necessary for Him to take upon Himself the burden of the earth-life in order to become the Savior of the people of the earth.

The occult teachings inform us that during His sojourn abroad, Jesus was simply a teacher, with but a dim perception of His real mission. But gradually He began to experience periods of Illumination in which He recognized His real nature and the difference between Himself and other men. Then came to Him the conviction of the mighty work that lay before Him in the redemption of the race, and He began to see the necessity of entering into the Karmic circle of the race in order to carry out the plan. This came gradually, by slow degrees, and the final sacrifice was made only in the Wilderness after His Baptism by John.

In the Wilderness, after His long fast and His days of meditation, the way opened up for Him to take upon Himself the burden of the Karma of the earth people. In that scene of the most tremendous spiritual struggle that the earth has ever witnessed, Jesus deliberately bent His shoulders that the weight be placed upon His back. From that moment the earth-souls received a blessing far beyond the comprehension of the mind of the ordinary man. Into the Karma-bound circle came this mighty soul, animated by Pure Spirit, for the purpose of lifting a great portion of the burden, and of joining in the work of the actual unfoldment and redemption of the race.

For be it remembered that, being a free soul animated by Pure

Spirit, Jesus was A GOD—not a man, although inhabiting the fleshly garments of humanity. His power was superior to that of many of the high intelligences scattered throughout the universe, and playing important parts in the cosmic processes. Jesus was Pure Spirit incarnate in human form, with all the powers of a God. Although of course subordinate in expression to the Absolute—the Great Spirit of Spirit—He was in His essential nature the same in substance. Verily, as He Himself said, "I and the Father are One."

His youthful mind was not able to grasp the truth of His real nature, but as that human instrument became perfected by age and training, He realized the Truth and perceived His own Divinity.

But even a God, such as he, could not raise up the world from its burden of Karma, by acting from the outside. Under the Cosmic Laws, established by the Absolute, such work could be performed only from within the circle of earth-life. And so Jesus saw that to raise up Man, He must become a Man. That is, to help lift the earth's Karma, He must enter into it, and place Himself within its Circle of Influence. And this He did.

We wonder if our readers can realize, even faintly, just what this sacrifice meant? Think of a Pure Spirit—a Free Soul—so filled with the love for the race of men as to renounce deliberately, for aeons of time, total immunity from all mortal existence, and willingly to place itself under the burden of pain, woe, misery and sin which formed the earth-people's Karma. It was a thousand-fold greater sacrifice than would be that of a Man of the Highest spiritual and mental development—an Emerson, for example—who, in order to raise up the race of earth-worms, would deliberately place himself within the being and nature of the Group-Soul animating the race of earthworms, and then stay within its influence, striving ever upward and onward until finally, after aeons and aeons of time, he was able to bring up the earthworm Group Soul to the level of Man. Think of this, and then realize what a sacrifice Jesus made of Himself.

In the Wilderness, when Jesus took the final steps of renunciation and sacrifice, He at once passed within the circle of the Race Karma and laid Himself open to all the pain, misery, temptations and limitations of a Man. His power, of course, remained with Him, but He was no longer a God outside of the world-life, but an imprisoned God working from within the race, using His mighty power, but bound by the Karmic Law. He became open to influences from which previously He had been immune. For instance when He was "tempted" by the Devil of Personal Attainment, and urged to seek worldly glory and renown, He was tempted only because He had taken on the world's Karma and was subject to its laws. As a God, He would not have felt the temptation any more than a man would feel the temptation of the earthworm. But as a man He was subject to the desires and ambitions that perplex and "devil" the race. And according to the rule that the greater the mental development the greater the power of such temptation toward self-aggrandizement (because of the mind being able to see more clearly the opportunities), Jesus was subjected to a test that would have been impossible to an ordinary man.

Jesus, knowing full well that He had in His possession the power to manifest the things with which He was tempted, was compelled to fight off the temptation to place Himself at the head of the race as its ruler—as the King of the World. He was shown this picture to compare with the other whose last scene was Calvary—and He was called upon to feel the desire of the race for such things, even unto its highest degree. Imagine the desire for personal aggrandizement of all the world thought beating upon His mind demanding the expression which could be had through Him alone. And then imagine the struggle required to defeat this opposing power. Think of what the ordinary man has to meet and overcome to conquer the desire for Personal Aggrandizement—and then think of what the Master had to fight, with the focussed desire of the entire Race-Thought striving to express itself through Him! Truly the Sins of the World bore down upon Him with their mighty weight. And yet He knew that He had taken upon Himself this affliction by entering upon the Life of Man. And He met it like a Man of Men.

It was only by fixing His mind fully and firmly upon what He knew to be His Real Self—the Spirit Within His soul, and holding His mind "one-pointed" upon the fact—that He was able to fight the fight and conquer. Seeing the Truth, He could see the folly and illusion of all that the world had to offer, and He could put forth His mighty Will bidding the Tempter retire from the scene and from His mind. It was in this full knowledge of His Spirit—His Real Self—that He was able to rebuke the Tempter, saying, "Thou shalt not tempt the Lord, thy God!" He held fast to His realization of the God Within—the Spirit that was within Him and all men—and thus denied out of existence the power of the earth-things—the illusions of mortality—the maya of the race.

But not alone this and other weaknesses of man's mortal nature were constantly besieging the mind of the Master after He had taken upon Himself the Karma of the Earth. He had also taken upon Himself the mortal life consequent of the human frame which He inhabited. He must live, suffer and die—even as all men—and according to the law of mortality. And so He moved forward toward the end, knowing fully what lay before Him. He, a God, had taken upon Himself all these attributes of mortality, in order to be able to perform His work as the Redeemer and Savior of the race.

And so, He lived, and suffered and died—even as you and I. He drank the cup to the dregs, suffering as only such a finely organized mental nature could suffer. And, men, poor creatures, speak of His sufferings as terminating with the last breath upon the cross. Why, they only began there!

For know ye, that Jesus the Christ is still within the race of men, suffering their woes, paying with them their penalty, every day, every hour—yea, and must remain so throughout the ages, until finally the soul of every man, yea, even that of the last man; the most degraded man in the world, is fully cleansed of the Karmic taint, and thus fully "redeemed" and "saved." And within the soul of every man is found the Christ Principle, striving ever to elevate and lift up the individual toward that realization of the Real Self—and this is what "redemption" and "salvation" really means. Not a saving from hell-fire, but a saving from the fire of carnality, and mortality. Not a redemption from imaginary sins, but a redemption from the muck and mire of earth-life. The God within you is like the fabled Hindu god who descended into the body of a pig and then forgot Himself. It is to bring you to a realization that you are a god and not a pig, that Jesus, the Master, is working within your soul as the Christ Principle. Have you never heard His voice, crying from within your soul, "Come out—come out of your pig-nature and realize the god that you verily are!" It is this "recognition, realization and manifestation of the god within you" that constitutes "salvation" and "redemption."

The Occult Teachings tell us that Jesus, after His final disappearance from before the eyes of His apostles, passed on to the higher planes of the Astral World where He rapidly discarded all of His astral and mental vehicles which the soul had used in its manifestation. The Astral Body and its corresponding higher sheaths were cast off and discarded. That is, all except the very highest of all. Had He discarded every vestige of individual soul-existence His spirit would have immediately merged itself with the One Spirit—the Absolute—from which it had originally proceeded and Jesus, as an entity, would have disappeared entirely within the Ocean of the One Spirit. This highest state of all He had deliberately resigned until the passage of ages, in order that He might accomplish His work as the World-Savior.

He retained the highest vehicle—the Spiritual Mind in its highest shade of expression—in order that as an entity He might labor for the race. And so, He exists at this time—one in substance with the Father, but yet maintaining an apparently separate entity-existence. But this must be remembered, that Jesus, as Jesus the son of Mary and Joseph, no longer exists. When He cast off the lower vehicles of His personality, His personality disappeared. But His individuality persisted—that is, He is still HE, although His personality has disappeared, leaving Him—the real Him—existing as the CHRIST PRINCIPLE.

By the above statement, we mean that when a soul reaches the highest spiritual stage short of absolute absorption into the One Spirit, it is no longer a person, but exists as a principle. But that principle is not an inanimate mechanical force—it is a living, knowing, acting principle of life. This occult fact cannot be explained in the words of men, for no terms have been coined by which men can speak of it. It is only indirectly that we can hope to have even the advanced student grasp the fact.

Jesus exists today, as the Christ Principle which actually lives and acts, but which is not confined in a body of any kind, using the word "body" in its accustomed sense. As the Christ Principle or "The Christ" He is mingled with the life of the human race, and may be found immanent in the mind of every man, woman and child that has ever existed, does now exist, or will exist so long as Man is Man. Not only is this true of those who have lived since His passage from the physical body, but it is equally true of those who lived before His birth. This apparently paradoxical statement may be understood when we remember that these souls did not "die," but only "passed on" to the Astral Plane, from whence they re-incarnated in due time. The Christ (for so we shall speak of the present-state of Jesus) even entered into, and still abides in, the Astral Plane, as well as upon the Material Plane, for wherever the souls of men abide—or whatever place their residence may be—there is found The Christ, ever working for the salvation and redemption of the race.

On the Astral Plane He is working in the minds of the souls abiding there, urging them to cast off the dross of earth-desires and to fix the aim upon higher things, to the end that their re-incarnations may be under improved conditions. On the Physical Plane He is working in the hearts and minds of the earth-people, striving ever to uplift to higher things. His aim is ever toward the liberation of the Spirit from its material bonds—the Realization of the Real Self. And so, in the hearts of all men, Christ is living, suffering, and being crucified every day, and this must continue until Man is redeemed and saved, even the last man.

This wonderful sacrifice of Christ far surpasses the physical sacrifice of Jesus, the man. Try to imagine, if you can, even the faintest pangs of a being so exalted compelled to dwell in the world of the hearts and minds of a humanity so steeped in materiality as our race, knowing always the possibilities of the souls if they would but reach upward to higher things, and yet constantly suffering the knowledge of the base, carnal, material thoughts and acts flowing from these souls. Is not this the extreme refinement of torture? Does not the agony of the cross sink into insignificance beside such spiritual agony? You rail at the cruelty of the Jews who crucified their Savior, and yet you crucify your Savior, with a thousandfold degree of torture, every day of your life, by your persistence in the carnalities and foolishness of mortal thought and action.

The mighty uplift of the world since the death of Jesus, of which the present is but a faint prophecy of the future, has been due largely to the energizing influence of The Christ in the hearts and minds of the race. The sense of the Fatherhood of God and the Brotherhood of Man, which is now manifesting so powerfully in the world of Men, is but an instance of the work of the Christ—the Savior and Redeemer. And the highest dreams of the exalted souls of this generation are but inadequate visions of what the future will hold for the race. The work is just beginning to bud—the blossom and the fruit will render this earth a far more glorious place than even the highest ideals of heaven entertained by the faithful in the past. But even these things of the future will be poor things, when compared with the life of the higher planes which await the race when it has demonstrated its fitness to pass on and on and on to these greater glories. And ever and ever The Christ is working, and toiling and striving and suffering, in His efforts to raise humanity even one petty degree in the spiritual scale of being.

The Christ is always with us, and if we but recognize His presence we shall be able to feel that warm, loving response to our soul-hunger and spiritual thirst which will result in our being given that we are so longingly craving. Here within us dwells The Christ, ever responding to the cry of Faith, "Believe in Me and ye shall be saved." What a promise this is seen to be when properly understood! What a source of power and comfort is opened up to every human soul when the Inner Truth underlying the teachings is understood! Mystic Christianity brings this Message of Truth to each and all of you who read these lines. Will you accept it?

We would ask our students to pause at this point and contrast the teachings of Mystic Christianity regarding the doctrine of Christ, the Savior, with the corresponding teachings of the current Orthodox Theology.

On the one hand we have Jesus the God-Man deliberately choosing the work of the World Redemption and Salvation, and descending into the circle of the World-Karma, relinquishing the privilege of His Godhood and taking upon Himself the penalties of Manhood; not only undergoing the sufferings of the physical man, but also binding Himself upon the Cross of Humanity for ages, that by His spiritual presence in and of the race He might lift up humanity to godhood.

On the other hand, we have a picture of an angry Deity, manifesting purely human emotion and temper, bent on revenging himself upon the race which he had created, and demanding its eternal punishment in hell-fire; then the same Deity creating a Son whom he sent into the world, that this Son might be the victim of a blood-atonement and death upon the cross, that the Deity's wrath might be appeased and the blood of this Divine Lamb be accepted to wash out the sins of the world.

Can you not see which is The Truth and which is the perversion? The one is from the pure fountain of Spiritual knowledge—the other originated in the minds of ignorant theologians who were unable to grasp and understand the Mystic teachings, but who built up a system of theology in accordance with their own undeveloped minds; making a God who was but a reflection of their own cruel animal natures, demanding, as did they themselves, blood and pain—physical torture and death—in order to appease a most un-Divine wrath and vengeance. Which of the two conceptions seems most in accord with the intuitive promptings of the Something Within? Which brings the greater approval from The Christ within your heart?

THE CHRISTIAN CREED

There are three creeds recognized by the Christian Church—the Apostles' Creed, the Nicene Creed, and the Athanasian Creed. Of these, the first two are commonly used, the third being not so well known and being seldom used.

The Apostles' Creed, which is the most commonly used, is believed (in its present form) to be of later origin than the Nicene Creed, and many authorities believe it to be a corrupted rendering of the original declaration of faith of the Early Christians. It is as follows:

> "I believe in God the Father Almighty, Maker of heaven and earth; and in Jesus Christ his only Son our Lord, who was conceived by the Holy Ghost, born of the Virgin Mary, suffered under Pontius Pilate, was crucified, dead and buried; he descended into hell; the third day he arose again from the dead; he ascended into heaven, and

sitteth on the right hand of God the Father Almighty; from thence he shall come to judge the quick and the dead. I believe in the Holy Ghost, the holy Catholic Church, the communion of saints, the forgiveness of sins, the resurrection of the body, and the life everlasting."

The Nicene Creed was drawn up and adopted by the Council of Nice in the year A.D. 325. As originally adopted it ended with the words "I believe in the Holy Ghost," the present concluding clauses being added by the Council of Constantinople in A.D. 381, excepting the words "and the Son," which were inserted by the Council of Toledo, A.D. 589. It is as follows:

"I believe in one God, the Father, Almighty, Maker of Heaven and earth, and all things visible and invisible; and in one Lord Jesus Christ, the only-begotten Son of God, begotten of his Father before all worlds, God of God, Light of Light, very God of very God, begotten, not made, being of one substance with the Father, by whom all things were made; who for us men and for our salvation came down from heaven and was incarnate by the Holy Ghost of the Virgin Mary, and was made man, and was crucified also for us under Pontius Pilate; he suffered and was buried and the third day he rose again according to the scriptures and ascended into heaven, and sitteth on the right hand of the Father; and he shall come again with glory to judge both the quick and the dead, whose kingdom shall have no end. And I believe in the Holy Ghost, the Lord and Giver of Life, who proceedeth from the Father and the Son, who with the Father and Son is worshipped and glorified, who spoke by the prophets; and I believe in one catholic and apostolic church; I acknowledge one baptism for the remission of sins, and I look for the resurrection of the dead and the life of the world to come."

Let us now briefly examine the principal statements of these creeds, which were compiled centuries after Jesus' death, viewing them by the light of Mystic Christianity.

"I believe in one God, the Father Almighty, Maker of heaven and earth, and all things visible and invisible."—(Nicene Creed.)

The form of the above fundamental principle of Christian belief is taken from the Nicene Creed, which is somewhat fuller than the similar declaration in the Apostles' Creed. It requires no comment. It is a statement of belief in a One Creative Power, from which all things have proceeded. There is no attempt made to "explain" the nature of the Absolute, or to endow it with any of the human attributes which theologians have delighted in bestowing upon the One. It merely asserts a belief in the existence of One Supreme Being—which is all that is possible to man—all else is ignorant impertinence.

"And in Jesus Christ his only Son our Lord, who was conceived by the Holy Ghost."—(Apostles' Creed.)

"And in one Lord Jesus Christ, the only begotten Son of God, begotten of his Father before all worlds, God of God, Light of Light, very God of very God, begotten, not made, being of one substance with the Father."—(Nicene Creed.)

In this declaration, the belief in the Divinity of Jesus is made. The Apostles' Creed shows the cruder conception, rather inclining toward the perverted idea of the conception of the Virgin by the aid of the Holy Ghost, similar to the origin of the hero-gods of the different religions in which the father was one of the gods and the mother a woman. But the Nicene creed gives at least a strong hint of the mystic teachings. It speaks of Him as "begotten of his Father"—"begotten, not made." The expressions, "God of God; Light of Light; very God of very God," show the idea of identical spiritual substance in the Spirit. And then the remarkable expression, "being of one substance with the Father," shows a wonderful understanding of the Mystery of The Christ. For, as the mystic teachings show, Jesus was a pure Spirit, free from the entangling desires and clogging Karma of the world. Identical in substance with the Father. "The Father and I are one," as He said. Is there anything in the Orthodox Theology that throws such light on this subject as is shed by Mystic Christianity's teaching regarding the nature of the soul of Jesus?

"Born of the Virgin Mary."—(Apostles' Creed.)

"Who for us men and for our salvation came down from heaven, and was incarnate by the Holy Ghost of the Virgin Mary, and was made man."—(Nicene Creed.)

The Nicene Creed here gives a surprisingly clear statement of the Mystic teachings. "Who for us men and our salvation came down from heaven" shows the purpose of the incarnation. "Came down from heaven" shows pre-existence in the bosom of the Absolute. "And was incarnate" shows the descent of the Spirit into the flesh in the womb of Mary. "And was made man" shows the taking on of the physical body of the infant in the womb. Does not the Mystic teaching give a clearer light on this statement of the Creed?

"Was crucified, dead and buried; he descended into hell; the third day he rose again from the dead."—(Apostles' Creed.)

"He suffered and was buried, and the third day he rose again according to the scriptures, and sitteth on the right hand of the Father."—(Nicene Creed.)

The "descent into hell" of the Apostles' Creed of course meant the passing to the place of disembodied souls—the lower Astral Plane. Even the orthodox teachers do not now pretend that the term "hell" meant the place of torture presided over by the Devil, which theology has invented to frighten people into the churches. "The third day he arose from the dead" (and the corresponding passage in the Nicene Creed) refers to the appearance in the Astral Body—the return from the Astral Plane in which He had sojourned for the three days following the crucifixion. "And ascended into heaven"—this passage shows the belief that He returned to the place from which He came, for the Nicene Creed has stated that he "came down from heaven and was incarnate ... and was made man."

The passage in both creeds stating that He then took his place "on the right hand of the Father" is intended to show that He took the place of the highest honor in the gift of the Father. The mystic teachings explain this by showing that The Christ is separated from The Father by but the most ethereal intervening of spiritual substance, and that He is a Cosmic Principle second in importance only to the Father. Truly this is the place of honor on "the right hand of the Father."

"He shall come to fudge the quick and the dead."

In this passage we see the intimation that not only with the "quick" or living people is The Christ concerned, but also with the "dead," that is, with those who "passed out" before and after His time and who have passed on to the Astral World, as we have explained in this lesson. Whether or not the framers of the Creed so understood it—whether or not they were deluded by the tradition of the "Day of Judgment"—certainly the Early Christians, or rather, the mystics among them, understood the teachings as we have given them and spoke of Him as "living in the dead as well as in the living," as one of the occult records expresses it.

"The communion of saints" is the spiritual understanding of the Mysteries by the Illumined Ones. "The forgiveness of sins" is the overcoming of the carnal mind and desires. "The resurrection of the dead and the life of the world to come" is the promise of life beyond the grave, and not the crude idea of the physical resurrection of the body, which has crept into the Apostles' Creed, evidently having been inserted at a later date in order to bolster up the pet theories of a school of theologians. Note that the Nicene Creed says merely "the dead" and not "the body." The version of the teachings preserved by the Mystics has a corresponding passage, "And we know the truth of the deathlessness of the soul." (The italics are ours.)

The consideration of remaining passages in the creeds, relating to the existence of the "Holy Ghost," must be deferred until our next lesson.

THE TENTH LESSON

THE SECRET DOCTRINE

The concluding statement of the Creeds (brought over from the preceding lesson) refers to the Holy Ghost.

"I believe in the Holy Ghost." (*Apostles' Creed.*)

"And I believe in the Holy Ghost, the Lord and giver of life." (*Nicene Creed.*)

To the average Christian the nature of the Holy Ghost—one of the beings of the Trinity—is veiled in obscurity, and is generally pronounced "not to be understood." A careful examination of the orthodox Christian writings will show the student that the Church is very much at sea regarding this subject, which should be of the greatest importance to its priests and congregations. Ask the average intelligent churchman regarding the nature of the Holy Ghost, and see for yourself the vague, contradictory and unsatisfactory concepts held by the person questioned. Then turn to the encyclopaedias and other books of reference, and see how little is known or taught regarding this important subject.

It is only when the teachings of Mystic Christianity are consulted that one receives any light on the subject. The Occult Teachings are quite explicit on this subject so fraught with difficulty and lack of comprehension on the part of the orthodox teachers and students.

The teaching of Mystic Christianity, regarding the Holy Ghost, may be summed up by the great general statement that: *The Holy Ghost is the Absolute in its phase of Manifestation, as compared to its phase of Unmanifestation—Manifest Being as compared with Unmanifest Being—God Create as compared with God Uncreate—God acting as the Creative Principle as compared to God as The Absolute Being.*

The student is asked to read over the above general statement a number of times and to concentrate his or her attention carefully upon it, before proceeding further with the lesson.

To understand the above statement it is necessary for the student to remember that the Absolute may be thought of as existing in two phases. Not as two persons or beings, remember, but as in two phases. There is but One Being—there can be but One—but we may think of that One as existing in two phases. One of these phases is Being Unmanifest; the other, Being Manifest.

Being Unmanifest is the One in its phase of Absolute Being,

undifferentiated, unmanifested, uncreated; without attributes, qualities, or natures.

It is impossible for the human mind to grasp the above concept of Being Manifest in the sense of being able to think of it as a "Thing, or Something." This because of the essential being of it. If it were like anything that we can think of, it would not be the Absolute, nor would it be Unmanifest. Everything that we can think of as a "thing" is a relative thing—a manifestation into objective being.

But we are compelled by the very laws of our reason to admit that the Absolute Being Unmanifest exists, for the Manifest and Relative Universe and Life must have proceeded and emanated from a Fundamental Reality, which must be Absolute and Unmanifest. And this Being which our highest reason causes us to assume to exist is Being Unmanifest—God the Father—who cannot be known through the senses—whose existence is made known to us only through Pure Reason, or through the workings of the Spirit within us. In the material sense "God is Unknowable"—but in the higher sense He may be known to the Spirit of Man, and His existence may be known and proven by the exercise of the highest faculties of the reason.

Being Unmanifest is the One in its actual existence and being. If all the world of objective life and manifestation, even to its highest forms, were withdrawn from manifestation, then there would be left—what? Simply and solely, Being Unmanifest—God the Father, alone. Into His Being all else would be withdrawn. Outside of Him there would be nothing. He would be Himself—One—existing in the phase of Being Unmanifest.

We are aware that this idea may seem to be "too abstruse" for the minds of some of our students at first reading—it may appear like an assertion of a Being who is Non-Being. But, be not too hasty—take time—and your mind will assimilate the concept, and will find that it has a corresponding Truth imbedded in its inmost recesses, and then it will know this to be the Truth. And then will it recognize the existence of God the Father, as compared with God, the Holy Ghost.

The Holy Ghost, as we have said, is the Absolute in its phase of Manifest Being. That is, it is God as manifest in the Spirit of Life, which is immanent in, and manifest in, all objective life and phenomena in the Cosmos or Universe.

In previous series of lessons in the Yogi Philosophy, we have shown you that there was a Spirit of Life immanent in, and manifesting through, all forms of life. We have also shown you that everything in the Universe is alive—down to even the minerals, and the atoms composing matter. We have shown you that inasmuch as the Spirit of Life is the source of all Manifestations in the universe, and the "God in the machine" of all phenomena of force, matter and life, then it naturally follows that there can be nothing dead in the world—that there is LIFE manifesting in every object, varying only in the degree of manifestation. In our "Advanced Lessons" and in "Gnani Yoga" this subject is considered in detail. Then what is this Spirit of Life? If God is All, then it cannot be Something other than God. But it cannot well be God the Uncreate—the Absolute in its Absolute phase—the Being Unmanifest. Then what can it be?

The student will see that the natural and logical answer to the question with which we have closed the preceding paragraph must be: Being Manifest—God in Creation—the Holy Ghost! And this is the Occult Teaching concerning this great mystery of Christianity. And see how well the framers of the Nicene Creed grasped the traditions of the Early Church, when it said: "And I believe in the Holy Ghost, the Lord and Giver of Life."

The teaching regarding the Immanent God lies at the foundation of all of the Mystic teachings of all peoples, races, and times. No matter under what names the teaching is promulgated—no matter what the name of the creed or religion in which it is found imbedded—it is still the Truth regarding the God Immanent in all forms of life, force, and matter. And it always is found forming the Secret Doctrine of the philosophy, creed or religion. The Outer Teaching generally confines itself to the instruction of the undeveloped minds of the people, and cloaks the real Truth behind some conception of a Personal Deity, or Deities—gods and demi-gods, who are supposed to dwell afar off in some heavenly realm—some great Being who created the world and then left it to run itself, giving it but occasional attention, and reserving his consideration principally for the purpose of rewarding those who gave him homage, worship and sacrifices and punishing those who failed to conform with the said requirements. These personal deities are believed generally to favor the particular people who give them their names and temples, and accordingly to hate the enemies of the said tribe or nation.

But the Secret Doctrine or Esoteric Teaching of all religions has brushed aside these primitive conceptions of undeveloped minds, and teach the Truth of the Immanent God—the Power inherent in and abiding in all life and manifestations. And Christianity is no exception to the rule, and in its declaration of faith in the Holy Ghost its esoteric principle is stated.

While the tendency of the orthodox churches today is to say very little about God the Holy Ghost, for the reason that it cannot explain the meaning of the term, Mystic Christianity boldly declares its allegiance to this principle of the earlier teachings and reverently repeats the words of the Nicene Creed, "I believe in the Holy Ghost, THE LORD AND GIVER OF LIFE."

* * * * *

That there is a Secret Doctrine of Christianity is not generally known to the majority who claim the name of "Christian." But it has always been known to the mystics in and out of the church, and its flame has been kept steadily alight by a few devoted souls who were chosen for this sacred task.

The Secret Doctrine of Christianity did not originate with Jesus, for He, Himself, was an Initiate of Mysteries which had been known and taught for centuries before His birth. As St. Augustine has said:

"That which is called the Christian Religion existed among the ancients and never did not exist, from the beginning of the human race until Christ came in the flesh, at which time the true religion which already existed began to be called Christianity."

We would like to quote here a few paragraphs from the writings of a well known writer on religious subjects, with which statement we heartily agree, although our views on certain other points of teaching do not agree with those of this writer. He says:

"It may be said that in the present day these doctrines are simply not taught in the churches; how is that? It is because Christianity has forgotten much of its original teachings, because it is now satisfied with only part, and a very small part, of what it originally knew. 'They still have the same scriptures,' you will say. Yes, but those very scriptures tell you often of something more, which is now lost. What is meant by Christ's constant references to the 'Mysteries of the Kingdom of God'—by His frequent statement to His disciples that the full and true interpretation could be given only to them, and that to others He must speak in parables? Why does He perpetually use the technical terms connected with the well known mystery-teaching of antiquity? What does St. Paul mean when he says, 'We speak wisdom among them which are perfect'—a well known technical term for the men at a certain stage of initiation? Again and again he uses terms of the same sort; he speaks of 'the wisdom of God in mystery, the hidden wisdom which God ordained before the world began, and which none even of the princes of this world know'—a statement which could not by any possibility have been truthfully made if he had been referring merely to ordinary Christian teaching which is openly preached before all men. His immediate followers, the Fathers of the Church, knew perfectly well what he meant, for they all use precisely the same phraseology. Clement of Alexandria, one of the earliest and greatest of all, tells us that 'It is not lawful to reveal to the profane persons the Mysteries of the Word.'"

"Another consideration shows us clearly how much of this early teaching has been lost. The church now devotes herself solely to producing good men, and points to the saint as her crowning glory and achievement. But in older days she claimed to be able to do much more than that. When she had made a man a saint, her work with him was only just beginning, for then only was he fit for the training and teaching which she could give him then, but cannot now, because she has forgotten her ancient knowledge. Then she had three definite stages in her course of training—Purification, Illumination and Perfection. Now she contents herself with the preliminary Purification, and has no Illumination to give."

"Read what Clement says: 'Purity is only a negative state, valuable chiefly as the condition of insight. He who has been purified in Baptism and then initiated into the Little Mysteries (has acquired, that is to say, the habits of self-control and reflection) becomes rife for the Greater Mysteries for the Gnosis, the scientific knowledge of God.' In another place he says: 'Knowledge is more than faith. Faith is a summary knowledge of urgent truths, suitable for people who are in a hurry; but knowledge is scientific faith.' And his pupil Origen writes of 'the popular, irrational faith' which leads to what he calls physical Christianity, based upon the gospel history, as opposed to the spiritual Christianity conferred by the Gnosis of Wisdom. Speaking of teaching founded upon historical narrative, he says, 'What better method could be devised to assist the masses?' But for those who are wise he has always the higher teachings, which are given only to those who have proved themselves worthy of it. This teaching is not lost; the church cast it out when she expelled the great Gnostic Doctors, but it has nevertheless been preserved, and it is precisely that Wisdom which we are studying—precisely that which we find to answer all the problems of life, to give us a rational rule by which to live, to be to us a veritable gospel of good news from on high."

St. Paul indicates the existence of the Secret Doctrine of Christianity, when he says to the Corinthians:

"And I, brethren, could not speak unto you as unto spiritual, but as unto carnal, as unto babes in Christ. I fed you with milk, not with meat; for ye were not yet able to bear it; nay, not even now are ye able, for ye are yet carnal." (I Cor. 3:1.)

Jesus said: "Give not that which is holy unto the dogs, neither cast your pearls before the swine, lest haply they trample them under their feet, and turn and rend you." (Matt. 7:6.)

St. Clement of Alexandria has said regarding the above saying of Jesus:

"Even now I fear, as it is said, 'to cast the pearls before swine, lest they tread them underfoot, and turn and rend us.' For it is difficult to exhibit the really pure and transparent words respecting the true Light to swinish and untrained hearers."

In the first century after Christ, the term "The Mysteries of Jesus" was frequently used by the Christian teachers, and the Inner Circle of Christians was recognized as a body of advanced souls who had developed so far as to be able to comprehend these mysteries.

The following passage from St. Mark (4:10-12) is interesting in this connection:

"And when He was alone, they that were about Him with the twelve asked of Him the parables. And He said unto them, 'Unto you is given the mystery of the kingdom of God: but unto them that are without, all things are done in parables: that seeing they may see, and not perceive; and hearing they may hear, and not understand.'"

The same writer says (4:33-34):

"And with many such parables spake He the word unto them, as they were able to hear it; and without a parable spake He not unto them; but privately to His own disciples He expounded all things."

Jesus said to His disciples (John 16:12.): "I have yet many things to say to you, but ye cannot bear them now." The Occult Teachings state that when He returned in His astral form, after the crucifixion, He taught them many important and advanced mystic truths, "speaking of the things pertaining to the kingdom of God." (Acts 1:3.)

The early Christian Fathers spake and wrote openly regarding the Christian Mysteries, as all students of Church History well know. Polycarp, Bishop of Smyrna, writes to certain others hoping that they are "well versed in the sacred Scriptures and that nothing is hidden from you; but to me this privilege is not yet granted." (The Epistle of Polycarp, chapter 7.) Ignatius, Bishop of Antioch, says that he is "not yet perfect in Jesus Christ. For I now begin to be a disciple, and I speak to you as my fellow disciple." He also addresses them as being "initiated into the Mysteries of the Gospel, with St. Paul, the holy, the martyred." Again:

"Might I not write to you things more full of mystery? But I fear to do so, lest I should inflict injury on you who are but babes. Pardon me in this respect, lest, as not being able to receive their weighty import, ye should be strangled by them. For even I, though I am bound and am able to understand heavenly things, the angelic orders, and the different sorts of angels and hosts, the distinction between powers and dominions, and the diversities between thrones and authorities, the mightiness of the aeons, and the preëminence of the cherubim and seraphim, the sublimity of the Spirit, the kingdom of the Lord, and above all the incomparable majesty of Almighty God—though I am acquainted with these things, yet am I not therefore by any means perfect, nor am I such a disciple as Paul or Peter."

Ignatius also speaks of the High Priest or Hierophant, of

whom he asserts that he was the one "to whom the holy of holies has been committed, and who alone has been entrusted with the secrets of God." (Epistles of Ignatius.)

St. Clement of Alexandria was a mystic of high rank in the Inner Circle of the Church. His writings are full of allusions to the Christian Mysteries. He says among other things that his writings were "a miscellany of Gnostic notes, according to the time philosophy," which teachings he had received from Pontaemus, his instructor or spiritual teacher. He says of these teachings:

"The Lord allowed us to communicate of those divine Mysteries and of that holy light, to those who are able to receive them. He did not certainly disclose to the many what did not belong to the many; but to the few to whom He knew that they belonged, who were capable of receiving and being moulded according to them. But secret things are intrusted to speech, not to writing, as is the case with God. And if one say that it is written, 'There is nothing secret which shall not be revealed, nor hidden, which shall not be disclosed,' let him also hear from us, that to him who hears secretly, even what is secret shall be manifested. This is what was predicted by this oracle. And to him who is able secretly to observe what is delivered to him, that which is veiled shall be disclosed as truth; and what is hidden to the many shall appear manifest to the few. The mysteries are delivered mystically, that what is spoken may be in the mouth of the speaker; rather not in his voice, but in his understanding. The writing of these memoranda of mine, I well know, is weak when compared with that spirit full of grace, which I was privileged to hear. But it will be an image to recall the archetype to him who was struck with the Thyrsus."

(We may state here that the Thyrsus was the mystic-wand carried by the Initiates in the Mystic Brotherhoods—the Initiate being first tapped with it, and then receiving it from the Hierophant, at the ceremony of formal Initiation.) Clement adds:

"We profess not to explain secret things sufficiently— far from it—but only to recall them to memory, whether we have forgot aught, or whether for the purpose of not forgetting. Many things, well I know, have escaped us, through length of time, that have dropped away unwritten. There are then some things of which we have no recollection; for the power that was in the blessed men was great."

"There are also some things which remain unnoted long, which have now escaped; and others which are effaced, having faded away in the mind itself, since such a task is not easy to those not experienced; these I revive in my commentaries. Some things I purposely omit, in the exercise of a wise selection, afraid to write what I guarded against speaking; not grudging—for that were wrong—but fearing for my readers lest they should stumble by taking them in a wrong sense; and, as the proverb says, we should be found 'reaching a sword to a child.' For it is impossible that what has been written should not escape, although remaining published by me. But being always revolved, using the one only voice, that of writing, they answer nothing to him that makes inquiries beyond what is written; for they require of necessity the aid of someone, either of him who wrote or of someone else, who walked in his footsteps. Some things my treatise will hint; on some it will linger; some it will merely mention. It will try to speak imperceptibly, to exhibit secretly, and to demonstrate silently." (The Stromata of St. Clement.)

St. Clement, in the same work from which the above quotation was taken, has a chapter entitled "The Mysteries of the Faith, not to be Divulged to all." In it he states that inasmuch as his writings might be seen by all men, the unwise as well as the wise, "it is requisite, therefore, to hide in a Mystery the wisdom spoken, in which the Son of God is taught." He then adds, "For it is difficult to exhibit the really pure and transparent words to swinish and untrained hearers. For scarcely could anything which they could bear be more ludicrous than these to the multitude; nor any subjects on the other hand more admirable or more inspiring to those of noble nature. But the wise do not utter with their mouths what they reason in council. 'But what ye hear in the ear,' said the Lord, 'proclaim upon the houses; bidding them receive the secret traditions of the true knowledge, and expound them aloft and conspicuously; and as we have said in the ear, so to deliver them to whom it is requisite; but not enjoining us to communicate to all without distinction what is said to them in parables. But there is only a delineation in the memoranda, which have the truth sown sparse and broadcast, that it may escape the notice of those who pick up seeds like jackdaws; but when they find a good husbandman, each of them will germinate and will produce corn."

"Those who are still blind and dumb, not having understanding, or the undazzled and keen vision of the contemplative soul, must stand outside of the divine choir. Wherefore, in accordance with the method of concealment, the truly sacred Word, truly divine and most necessary for us, deposited in the shrine of truth, was by the Egyptians indicated by what were called among them adyta, and by the Hebrews 'the veil.' Only the consecrated were allowed access to them. For Plato also thought it not lawful for 'the impure to touch the pure.' Thence the prophecies and oracles are spoken in enigmas, and to the untrained and uninstructed people. Now, then, it is not wished that all things should be exposed indiscriminately to all and sundry, or the benefits of wisdom communicated to those who have not even in a dream been purified in soul, for it is not allowable to hand to every chance comer what has been procured with such laborious efforts. Nor are the Mysteries of the Word to be expounded to the profane. The Mysteries were established for the reason that it was more beneficial that the holy and the blessed contemplation of realities be conceded. So that, on the other hand, then, there are the Mysteries which were hid till the time of the apostles, and were delivered by them as they received from the Lord, and, concealed in the Old Testament, were manifested to the saints. And on the other hand, there is the riches of the glory of the mysteries of the Gentiles, which is faith and hope in Christ. Instruction, which reveals hidden things, is called Illumination, as it is the teacher only who uncovers the lid of the ark." (The Stromata of St. Clement.)

St. Clement also quotes approvingly the saying of Plato, that: "We must speak in enigmas; that should the tablet come by any mischance on its leaves either by sea or land he who reads may remain ignorant." He also says, concerning certain Gnostic writings:

"Let the specimen suffice to those who have ears. For it is not required to unfold the mystery, but only to indicate what is sufficient for those who are partakers in knowledge to bring it to mind."

We have quoted freely from St. Clement, for the purpose of showing that he, a man in a very exalted position in the Early Christian Church, recognized, and actually taught, the Inner Teachings, or Secret Doctrine of Mystic Christianity—that the Early Christian Church was an organization having a Mystic Centre for the few, and Common Outer for the multitude. Can there be any doubt of this after reading the above words from his pen?

But not only St. Clement so wrote and taught, but many others in authority in the Early Christian Church likewise voiced their knowledge of, and approval in, the Inner Teachings. For example, Origen, the pupil of St. Clement, a man whose influence was felt on all sides in the early days of the Church. Origen defended Christianity from the attacks of Celsus, who charged the Church with being a secret organization which taught the Truth only to a few, while it satisfied the multitude with popular teachings and half-truths. Origen replied that, while it was true that there were Inner Teachings in the Church which were not revealed to the general public, still the Church, in that respect, was but following the example of all teachers of Truth, who always maintained an esoteric side of their teachings for those fitted to participate in them, while giving the exoteric side to the general body of followers. He writes:

"And yet the Mystery of the Resurrection, not being understood, is made a subject of ridicule among unbelievers. In these circumstances, to speak of the Christian doctrine as a secret system is altogether absurd. But that there should be certain doctrines, not made known to the multitude, which are divulged after the exoteric ones have been taught, is not a peculiarity of Christianity alone, but also of philosophic systems in which certain truths are exoteric and others esoteric. Some of the hearers of Pythagoras were content with his ipse dixit; while others were taught in secret those doctrines which were not deemed fit to be communicated to profane and insufficiently prepared ears. Moreover, all the Mysteries that are celebrated everywhere throughout Greece and barbarous countries, although held in secret, have no discredit thrown upon them, so that it is in vain he endeavors to calumniate the secret doctrines of Christianity, seeing that he does not correctly understand its nature."

"I have not yet spoken of the observance of all that is written in the Gospels, each one of which contains much doctrine difficult to be understood, not merely by the multitude, but even by certain of the more intelligent, including a very profound explanation of the parables, which Jesus delivered to 'those without' while reserving the exhibition of their full meaning for those who had passed beyond the stage of exoteric teaching, and who came to Him privately in the house. And when he comes to understand it, he will admire the reason why some are said to be 'without' and others 'in the house.'" (Origen against Celsus.)

In the same work Origen considers the story of the Syria-Phoenician woman (Matt. Chap. 15) and says concerning it:

"And perhaps, also, of the words of Jesus there are some loaves which it is possible to give to the more rational, as to the children, only; and others as it were crumbs from the great house and table of the well-born, which may be used by some souls like dogs."

And, again,

"He whose soul has, for a long time, been conscious of no evil, especially since he yielded himself to the healing of the Word, let such a one hear the doctrines which were spoken in private by Jesus to His genuine disciples."

And, again,

"But on these subjects much, and that of a mystical kind, might be said: in keeping with which is the following: 'It is good to keep close to the secret of a king,' in order that the doctrine of the entrance of souls into bodies may not be thrown before the common understanding, nor what is holy given to the dogs, nor pearls be cast before swine. For such a procedure would be impious, being equivalent to a betrayal of the mysterious declaration of God's wisdom. It is sufficient, however, to represent in the style of a historic narrative what is intended to convey a secret meaning in the garb of history, that those who have the capacity may work out for themselves all that relates to the subject."

He also says, in the same work:

"If you come to the books written after the time of Jesus, you will find that those multitudes of believers who hear the parables are, as it were, 'without,' and worthy only of exoteric doctrines, while the disciples learn in private the explanation of the parables. For, privately, to His own disciples did Jesus open up all things, esteeming above the multitudes those who desired to know His wisdom. And He promises to those who believe on Him to send them wise men and scribes."

In another work, Origen states that:

"The Scriptures have a meaning, not only such as is apparent at first sight, but also another, which escapes the notice of most men. For such is written in the forms of certain Mysteries, and the image of divine things. Respecting which there is one opinion throughout the whole Church, that the whole law is indeed spiritual; but that the spiritual meaning which the law conveys is not known to all, but to those only on whom the grace of the Holy Spirit is bestowed in the word of wisdom and knowledge." (De Principiis.)

We could fill page after page with live quotations from the writings of the Early Christian Fathers, and their successors, showing the existence of the Inner Teachings. But we must rest content with those which we have given you, which are clear and to the point, and which come from undoubted authority.

The departure of the Church from these Inner Teachings was a great calamity, from which the Church is still suffering. As that well-known occultist, Eliphias Levi, has said:

"A great misfortune befell Christianity. The betrayal of the Mysteries by the false Gnostics—for the Gnostics, that is, those who know, were the Initiates of primitive Christianity—caused the Gnosis to be rejected, and alienated the Church from the supreme truths of the Kabbala, which contains all the secrets of transcendental theology.... Let the most absolute science, let the highest reason become once more the patrimony of the leaders of the people; let the sarcerdotal art and the royal art take the double sceptre of antique initiations and the social world will once more issue from its chaos. Burn the holy images no longer; demolish the temples no more; temples and images are necessary for men; but drive the hirelings from the house of prayer; let the blind be no longer leaders of the blind; reconstruct the hierarchy of intelligence and holiness, and recognize only those who know as the teachers of those who believe." (The Mysteries of Magic, Waite translation.)

And now, you ask, what were taught in these Christian Mysteries—what is the Inner Teaching—what the Secret Doctrine? Simply this, good students—the Occult Philosophy and Mystic Lore which has been taught to the Elect in all times and ages, and which is embodied in our several series of lessons on THE YOGI PHILOSOPHY AND ORIENTAL OCCULTISM, plus the special teaching regarding the nature, mission, and sacrifice of Jesus the Christ, as we have tried to explain in the present series of lessons. The Truth is the same no matter under what name it is taught, or who teaches it. Strip it of the personal coloring of the teacher and it is seen to be the same—THE TRUTH.

In these lessons we have tried to give you the Key to the Mysteries, but unless you have studied the other lessons in which the Occult Teachings have been set forth, you will not be able to see their application in Mystic Christianity. You must bring Knowledge to these lessons, in order to take away knowledge.

THE ELEVENTH LESSON

THE ANCIENT WISDOM

The doctrine of Metempsychosis or Re-incarnation has its roots deeply imbedded in the soil of all religions—that is, in the Inner Teachings or Esoteric phase of all religious systems. And this is true of the Inner Teachings of the Christian Church as well as of the other systems. The Christian Mysteries comprised this as well as the other fundamental occult doctrines, and the Early Church held such teachings in its Inner Circle.

And, in its essence, the doctrine of Re-birth is the only one that is in full accord with the Christian conception of ultimate justice and "fairness." As a well known writer has said concerning this subject:

> "It relieves us of many and great difficulties. It is impossible for any one who looks around him and sees the sorrow and suffering in the world, and the horrible inequality in the lives of men—not inequality in wealth merely, but inequality in opportunity of progress—to harmonize these facts with the love and justice of God, unless he is willing to accept this theory that this one life is not all, but that it is only a day in the real life of the soul, and that each soul therefore has made its place for itself, and is receiving just such training as is best for its evolution. Surely the only theory which enables a man rationally to believe in Divine justice, without shutting his eyes to obvious facts, is a theory worthy of study.
>
> "Modern theology concerns itself principally with a plan for evading divine justice, which it elects to call 'Salvation,' and it makes this plan depend entirely upon what a man believes, or rather upon what he says that he believes. This whole theory of 'salvation,' and indeed the theory that there is anything to be 'saved' from, seems to be based upon a misunderstanding of a few texts of scripture. We do not believe in this idea of a so-called divine wrath; we think that to attribute to God our own vices of anger and cruelty is a terrible blasphemy. We hold to the theory of steady evolution and final attainment for all; and we think that the man's progress depends not upon what he

believes, but upon what he does. And there is surely very much in the bible to support this idea. Do you remember St. Paul's remark, 'Be not deceived, God is not mocked; whatsoever a man soweth, that shall he also reap'? And again, Christ said that 'They that have done good shall go unto the resurrection of life'—not they that have believed some particular doctrine. And when He describes the day of judgment, you will notice that no question is raised as to what anybody has believed, but only as to the works which he has done."

In this connection, we think that it is advisable to quote from the address of a well known English churchman upon this important subject. The gentleman in question is The Ven. Archdeacon Colley, Rector of Stockton, Warwickshire, England, who said:

"In the realm of the occult and transcendental, moved to its exploration from the Sadducean bias of my early days, I have for the best part of half a century had experiences rarely equaled by any, and I am sure, surpassed by none; yet have they led me up till now, I admit, to no very definite conclusions. With suspension of judgment, therefore, not being given to dogmatize on anything, and with open mind I trust, in equipoise of thought desiring to hold an even balance of opinion 'twixt this and that, I am studious still of being receptive of light from every source—rejecting nothing that in the least degree makes for righteousness, hence my taking the chair here tonight, hoping to learn what may help to resolve a few of the many perplexities of life, to wit: Why some live to the ripe old age of my dear father while others live but for a moment, to be born, gasp and die. Why some are born rich and others poor; some having wealth only to corrupt, defile, deprave others therewith, while meritorious poverty struggles and toils for human betterment all unaided. Some gifted with mentality; others pitiably lacking capacity. Some royal-souled from the first naturally, others with brutal, criminal propensities from beginning to end.

"The sins of the fathers visited upon the children unto the third and fourth generation may in heredity account for much, but I want to see through the mystery of a good father at times having a bad son, as also of one showing genius and splendid faculties—the offspring of parentage the reverse of anything suggesting qualities contributive thereto. Then as a clergyman, I have in my reading noted texts of Holy Scripture, and come across passages in the writings of the Fathers of the Early Church which seem to be root-thoughts, or survivals of the old classic idea of re-incarnation.

"The prophet Jeremiah (1:5) writes, 'The word of the Lord came unto me saying, before I formed thee, I knew thee, and before thou wast born I sanctified thee and ordained thee a prophet.'

"Does this mean that the Eternal-Uncreate chose, from foreknowledge of what Jeremiah would be, the created Ego of His immaterialized servant in heaven ere he clothed his soul with the mortal integument of flesh in human birth—schooling him above for the part he had to play here below as a prophet to dramatize in his life and teaching the will of the Unseen? To the impotent man at the Pool of Bethesda, whose infirmity was the cruel experience of eight and thirty years, the Founder of our religion said (John 5:14.), 'Behold, thou art made whole; sin no more, lest a worse thing come unto thee.' Was it (fitting the punishment to the crime proportionately) some outrageous sin as a boy, in the spring of years and days of his inexperienced youth of bodily life, that brought on him such physical sorrow, which youthful sin in its repetition would necessitate an even worse ill than this nearly forty years of sore affliction? 'Who did sin, this man or his parents, that he was born blind?' (John 9:2.), was the question of the disciples to Jesus. And our query is—Sinned before he was born to deserve the penalty of being born blind?

"Then of John the Baptist—was he a reincarnation of Elijah, the prophet, who was to come again? (Malachi 4:5.). Jesus said he was Elijah, who indeed had come, and the evil-minded Jews had done unto him whatsoever they listed. Herod had beheaded him (Matt. 11:14 and 17:12.).

"Elijah and John the Baptist appear from our reference Bibles and Cruden's Concordance to concur and commingle in one. The eighth verse of the first chapter of the second Book of Kings and the fourth verse of the third chapter of St. Matthew's Gospel note similarities in them and peculiarities of dress. Elijah, as we read, was a 'hairy man and girt a leathern girdle about his loins,' while John the Baptist had 'his raiment of camel's hair and a leathern girdle about his loins.' Their home was the solitude of the desert. Elijah journeyed forty days and forty nights unto Horeb, the mount of God in the Wilderness of Sinai. John the Baptist was in the wilderness of Judea beyond Jordan baptizing. And their life in exile—a self-renunciating and voluntary withdrawal from the haunts of men—was sustained in a parallel remarkable way by food (bird—brought on wing—borne). 'I have commanded the ravens to feed thee,' said the voice of Divinity to the prophet; while locusts and wild honey were the food of the Baptist.

"'And above all,' said our Lord of John the Baptist to the disciples, 'if ye will receive it, this is Elias which was for to come.'

"Origen, in the second century, one of the most learned of the Fathers of the early Church, says that this declares the pre-existence of John the Baptist as Elijah before his decreed later existence as Christ's forerunner.

"Origen also says on the text, 'Jacob I have loved, but Esau I have hated,' that if our course be not marked out according to our works before this present life that now is, how would it not be untrue and unjust in God that the elder brother should serve the younger and be hated by God (though blessed of righteous Abraham's son, of Isaac) before Esau had done anything deserving of servitude or given any occasion for the merciful Almighty's hatred?

"Further, on the text (Ephesians 1:4.), 'God who hath chosen us before the foundation of the world,' Origen says that this suggests our pre-existence ere the world was.

"While Jerome, agreeing with Origen, speaks of our rest above, where rational creatures dwell before their descent to this lower world, and prior to their removal from the invisible life of the spiritual sphere to the visible life here on earth, teaching, as he says, the necessity of their again having material bodies ere, as saints and men made 'perfect as our Father which is in heaven is perfect,' they once more enjoy in the angel-world their former blessedness.

"Justin Martyr also speaks of the soul inhabiting the human body more than once, but thinks as a rule (instanced in the case of John the Baptist forgetting that he had been Elijah) it is not permitted us to remember our former experiences of this life while yet again we are in exile here as strangers and pilgrims in an uncongenial clime away from our heavenly home.

"Clemens Alexandrinus, and others of the Fathers, refer to reincarnation (or transmigration or metempsychosis, as it is called in the years that are passed of classic times and later now as re-birth) to remind us of the vital truth taught by our Lord in the words, 'Ye must be born again.'"

These words, falling from the lips of a man so eminent in the staid conservative ranks of the Church of England, must attract the attention of every earnest seeker after the Truth of Christian Doctrine. If such a man, reared in such an environment, could find himself able to bear such eloquent testimony to the truth of a philosophy usually deemed foreign to his accepted creed, what might we not expect from a Church liberated from the narrow formal bounds of orthodoxy, and once more free to consider, learn and teach those noble doctrines originally held and taught by the Early Fathers of the Church of Christ?

While the majority of modern Christians bitterly oppose the idea that the doctrine of Metempsychosis ever formed any part of the Christian Doctrine, and prefer to regard it as a "heathenish" teaching, still the fact remains that the careful and unprejudiced student will find indisputable evidence in the writings of the Early Christian Fathers pointing surely to the conclusion that the doctrine of Metempsychosis was believed and taught in the Inner Circle of the Early Church.

The doctrine unquestionably formed a part of the Christian Mysteries, and has faded into comparative obscurity with the decay of spirituality in the Church, until now the average churchman no longer holds to it, and in fact regards as barbarous and heathenish that part of the teachings originally imparted and taught by the Early Fathers of the Church—the Saints and Leaders.

The Early Christians were somewhat divided in their beliefs concerning the details of Re-birth. One sect or body held to the idea that the soul of man was eternal, coming from the Father. Also that there were many degrees and kinds of souls, some of which have never incarnated in human bodies but which are living on many planes of life unknown to us, passing from plane to plane, world to world. This sect held that some of these souls had chosen to experiment with life on the physical plane, and were now passing through the various stages of the physical-plane life, with all of its pains and sorrows, being held by the Law of Re-birth until a full experience had been gained, when they would pass out of the circle of influence of the physical plane, and return to their original freedom.

Another sect held to the more scientific occult form of the gradual evolution of the soul, by repeated rebirth, on the physical plane, from Lower to Higher, as we have set forth in our lessons on "Gnani Yoga." The difference in the teachings arose from the different conceptions of the great leaders, some being influenced by the Jewish Occult Teachings which held to the first above mentioned doctrine, while the second school held to the doctrine taught by the Greek Mystics and the Hindu Occultists. And each interpreted the Inner Teachings by the light of his previous affiliations.

And so, some of the early writings speak of "pre-existence," while others speak of repeated "rebirth." But the underlying principle is the same, and in a sense they were both right, as the advanced occultists know full well. The fundamental principle of both conceptions is that the soul comes forth as an emanation from the Father in the shape of Spirit; that the Spirit becomes plunged in the confining sheaths of Matter, and is then known as "a soul," losing for a time its pristine purity; that the soul passes on through rebirth, from lower to higher, gaining fresh experiences at each incarnation; that the advancing soul passes from world to world, returning at last to its home laden with the varied experiences of life and becomes once more pure Spirit.

The early Christian Fathers became involved in a bitter controversy with the Greek and Roman philosophers, over the conception held by some of the latter concerning the absurd doctrine of the transmigration of the human soul into the body of an animal. The Fathers of the Church fought this erroneous teaching with great energy, their arguments bringing out forcibly the distinction between the true occult teachings and this erroneous and degenerate perversion in the doctrines of transmigration into animal bodies. This conflict caused a vigorous denunciation of the teachings of the Pythagorean and Platonic schools, which held to the perverted doctrine that a human soul could degenerate into the state of the animal.

Among other passages quoted by Origen and Jerome to prove the pre-existence of the soul was that from Jeremiah (1:5): "Before thou comest from the womb I sanctified thee and I ordained thee a prophet." The early writers held that this passage confirmed their particular views regarding the pre-existence of the soul and the possession of certain characteristics and qualities acquired during previous birth, for, they argued, it would be injustice that a man, before birth, be endowed with uncarnal qualities; and that such qualities and ability could justly be the result only of best work and action. They also dwelt upon the prophecy of the return of Elijah, in Malachi 4:5. And also upon the (uncanonical) book "The Wisdom of Solomon," in which Solomon says: "I was a witty child, and had a good Spirit. Yea, rather, being good, I came into a body undefiled."

They also quoted from Josephus, in his book styled "De Bello Judico," in which the eminent Jewish writer says: "They say that all souls are incorruptible; but that the souls of good men are only removed into other bodies—but that the souls of bad men are subject to eternal punishment." They also quoted from Josephus, regarding the Jewish belief in Rebirth as evidenced by the recital of the instance in which, at the siege of the fortress of Jotapota, he sought the shelter of a cave in which were a number of soldiers, who discussed the advisability of committing suicide for the purpose of avoiding being taken prisoners by the Romans. Josephus remonstrated with them as follows:

> "Do ye not remember that all pure spirits who are in conformity with the divine dispensation live on in the loveliest of heavenly places, and in the course of time they are sent down to inhabit sinless bodies; but the souls of those who have committed self-destruction are doomed to a region in the darkness of the underworld?"

Recent writers hold that this shows that he accepted the doctrine of Re-birth himself, and also as showing that it must have been familiar to the Jewish soldiery.

There seems to be no doubt regarding the familiarity of the Jewish people of that time with the general teachings regarding Metempsychosis. Philo positively states the doctrine as forming part of the teachings of the Jewish Alexandrian school. And again the question asked Jesus regarding the "sin of the man born blind" shows how familiar the people were with the general doctrine.

And so, the teachings of Jesus on that point did not need to be particularly emphasized to the common people, He reserving this instruction on the inner teachings regarding the details of Re-birth for his chosen disciples. But still the subject is mentioned in a number of places in the New Testament, as we shall see.

Jesus stated positively that John the Baptist was "Elias," whose return had been predicted by Malachi (4:5). Jesus stated this twice, positively, i.e., "This is Elijah that is to come" (Matt. 11:14); and again, "But I say unto you that Elijah is come already, but they knew him not, but did unto him whatsoever they would.... Then understood the disciples that he spoke unto them of John the Baptist." (Matt. 17:12-13.) The Mystics point out that Jesus saw clearly the fact that John was Elijah re-incarnated, although John had denied this fact, owing to his lack of memory of his past incarnation. Jesus the Master saw clearly that which John the Forerunner had failed to perceive concerning himself. The plainly perceptible characteristics of Elijah reappearing in John bear out the twice-repeated, positive assertion of the Master that John the Baptist was the re-incarnated Elijah.

And this surely is sufficient authority for Christians to accept the doctrine of Re-birth as having a place in the Church Teachings.

But still, the orthodox churchmen murmur "He meant something else!" There are none so blind as those who refuse to see.

Another notable instance of the recognition of the doctrine by Jesus and His disciples occurs in the case of "the man born blind." It may be well to quote the story.

> "And as he passed by he saw a man blind from his birth. And his disciples asked him, saying, 'Rabbi, who sinned, this man or his parents, that he should be born blind?' Jesus answered, 'Neither did this man sin nor his parents.'" (John 9:1-3.)

Surely there can be no mistake about the meaning of this question, "Who did sin, this man or his parents?"—for how could a man sin before his birth, unless he had lived in a previous incarnation? And the answer of Jesus simply states that the man was born blind neither from the sins of a past life, nor from those of his parents, but from a third cause. Had the idea of re-incarnation been repugnant to the teachings, would not He have denounced it to His disciples? Does not the fact that His disciples asked Him the question show that they were in the habit of discoursing the problems of Re-birth and Karma with Him, and receiving instructions and answers to questions propounded to Him along these lines?

There are many other passages of the New Testament which go to prove the familiarity of the disciples and followers of Jesus with the doctrine of Re-birth, but we prefer to pass on to a consideration of the writings of the Early Christian Fathers in order to show what they thought and taught regarding the matter of Re-birth and Karma.

Among the great authorities and writers in the Early Church, Origen stands out pre-eminently as a great light. Let us quote from a leading writer, regarding this man and his teachings:

> "In Origen's writings we have a mine of information as to the teachings of the early Christians. Origen held a splendid and grandiose view of the whole of the evolution of our system. I put it to you briefly. You can read it in all its carefully, logically-worked-out arguments, if you will have the patience to read his treatise for yourselves. His view, then, was the evolutionary view. He taught that forth from God came all Spirits that exist, all being dowered with free-will; that some of these refused to turn aside from the path of righteousness, and, as a reward, took the place

which we speak of as that of the angels; that then there came others who, in the exercise of their free-will, turned aside from the path of deity, and then passed into the human race to recover, by righteous and noble living, the angel condition which they had not been able to preserve; that others, still in the exercise of their free-will, descended still deeper into evil and became evil spirits or devils. So that all these Spirits were originally good; but good by innocence, not by knowledge. And he points out also that angels may become men, and even the evil ones themselves may climb up once more, and become men and angels again. Some of you will remember that one of the doctrines condemned in Origen in later days was that glorious doctrine that, even for the worst of men, redemption and restoration were possible, and that there was no such thing as an eternity of evil in a universe that came from the Eternal Goodness, and would return whence it came."

And from the writings of this great man we shall now quote.

In his great work "De Principiis," Origen begins with the statement that only God Himself is fundamentally and by virtue of His essential nature, Good. God is the only Good—the absolute perfect Good. When we consider the lesser stages of Good, we find that the Goodness is derived and acquired, instead of being fundamental and essential. Origen then says that God bestows free-will upon all spirits alike, and that if they do not use the same in the direction of righteousness, then they fall to lower estates "one more rapidly, another more slowly, one in a greater, another in a less degree, each being the cause of his own downfall."

He refers to John the Baptist being filled with the Holy Ghost in his mother's womb and says that it is a false notion to imagine "that God fills individuals with His Holy Spirit, and bestows upon them sanctification, not on the grounds of justice and according to their deserts, but undeservedly. And how shall we escape the declaration, 'Is there respect of persons with God?' God forbid. Or this, 'Is there unrighteousness with God?' God forbid this also. For such is the defense of those who maintain that souls come into existence with bodies." He then shows his belief in re-birth by arguing that John had earned the Divine favor by reason of right-living in a previous incarnation.

Then he considers the important question of the apparent injustice displayed in the matter of the inequalities existing among men. He says, "Some are barbarians, others Greeks, and of the barbarians some are savage and fierce and others of a milder disposition, and certain of them live under laws that have been thoroughly approved, others, again, under laws of a more common or severe kind; while, some, again, possess customs of an inhumane and savage character rather than laws; and certain of them, from the hour of their birth, are reduced to humiliation and subjection, and brought up as slaves, being placed under the dominion either of masters, or princes, or tyrants. Some with sound bodies, some with bodies diseased from their early years, some defective in vision, others in bearing and speech; some born in that condition, others deprived of the use of their senses immediately after birth. But why should I repeat and enumerate all the horrors of human misery? Why should this be?"

Origen then goes on to combat the ideas advanced by some thinkers of his times, that the differences were caused by some essential difference in the nature and quality of the souls of individuals. He states emphatically that all souls are essentially equal in nature and quality and that the differences arise from the various exercise of their power of free-will. He says of his opponents:

> "Their argument accordingly is this: If there be this great diversity of circumstances, and this diverse and varying condition by birth, in which the faculty of free-will has no scope (for no one chooses for himself either where, or with whom, or in what condition he is born); if, then, this is not caused by the difference in the nature of souls, i.e., that a soul of an evil nature is destined for a wicked nation and a good soul for a righteous nation, what other conclusion remains than that these things must be supposed to be regulated by accident or chance? And, if that be admitted, then it will be no longer believed that the world was made by God, or administered by His providence."

Origen continues:

> "God who deemed it just to arrange His creatures according to their merit, brought down these different understandings into the harmony of one world, that He might adorn, as it were, one dwelling, in which there ought to be not only vessels of gold and silver, but also of wood and clay (and some, indeed, to honor, and others to dishonor) with their different vessels, or souls, or understandings. On which account the Creator will neither

appear to be unjust in distributing (for the causes already mentioned) to every one according to his wants, nor will the happiness or unhappiness of each one's birth, or whatever be the condition that falls to his lot, be accidental."

He then asserts that the condition of each man is the result of his own deeds.

He then considers the case of Jacob and Esau, which a certain set of thinkers had used to illustrate the unjust and cruel discrimination of the Creator toward His creatures. Origen contended that in this case it would be most unjust for God to love Jacob and hate Esau before the children were born, and that the only true interpretation of the matter was the theory that Jacob was being rewarded for the good deeds of past lives, while Esau was being punished for his misdeeds in past incarnations.

And not only Origen takes this stand, but Jerome also, for the latter says: "If we examine the case of Esau we may find he was condemned because of his ancient sins in a worse course of life." (Jerome's letter to Avitus.) Origen says:

> "It is found not to be unrighteous that even in womb Jacob supplanted his brother, if we feel that he was worthily beloved by God, according to the deserts of his previous life, so as to deserve to be preferred before his brother."

Origen adds, "This must be carefully applied to the case of all other creatures, because, as we formerly remarked, the righteousness of the Creator ought to appear in everything." And again, "The inequality of circumstances preserves the justice of a retribution according to merit."

Annie Besant (to whom we are indebted for a number of these quotations), says, concerning this position of Origen:

> "Thus we find this doctrine made the defense of the justice of God. If a soul can be made good, then to make a soul evil is to a God of justice and love impossible. It cannot be done. There is no justification for it, and the moment you recognize that men are born criminal, you are either forced into the blasphemous position that a perfect and loving God creates a ruined soul and then punishes it for being what He has made it, or else that He is dealing with growing, developing creatures whom He is training

for ultimate blessedness, and if in any life a man is born wicked and evil, it is because he has done amiss and must reap in sorrow the results of evil in order that he may learn wisdom and turn to good."

Origen also considers the story of Pharaoh, of whom the Biblical writers say that "his heart was hardened by God." Origen declares that the hardening of the heart was caused by God so that Pharaoh would more readily learn the effect of evil, so that in his future incarnations he might profit by his bitter experience. He says:

"Sometimes it does not lead to good results for a man to be cured too quickly, especially if the disease, being shut up in the inner parts of the body, rage with greater fierceness. The growth of the soul must be understood as being brought about not suddenly, but slowly and gradually, seeing that the process of amendment and correction will take place imperceptibly in the individual instances, during the lapse of countless and unmeasured ages, some outstripping others, and tending by a swifter course towards perfection, while others, again, follow close at hand, and some, again, a long way behind."

He also says: "Those who, departing this life in virtue of that death which is common to all, are arranged in conformity with their actions and deserts—according as they shall be deemed worthy—some in the place called the 'infernus,' others in the bosom of Abraham, and in different localities or mansions. So also from these places, as if dying there, if the expression can be used, they come down from the 'upper world' to this 'hell.' For that 'hell' to which the souls of the dead are conducted from this world is, I believe, on account of this destruction, called 'the lower hell.' Everyone accordingly of those who descend to the earth is, according to his deserts, or agreeably to the position that he occupied there, ordained to be born in this world in a different country, or among a different nation, or in a different mode of life, or surrounded by infirmities of a different kind, or to be descended from religious parents, or parents who are not religious; so that it may sometimes happen that an Israelite descends among the Scythians, and a poor Egyptian is brought down to Judea." (Origen against Celsus.)

Can you doubt, after reading the above quotation that Metempsychosis, Re-incarnation or Re-birth and Karma was held and taught as a true doctrine by the Fathers of the Early Christian

Church? Can you not see that imbedded in the very bosom of the Early Church were the twin-doctrine of Re-incarnation and Karma. Then why persist in treating it as a thing imported from India, Egypt or Persia to disturb the peaceful slumber of the Christian Church? It is but the return home of a part of the original Inner Doctrine—so long an outcast from the home of its childhood.

The Teaching was rendered an outlaw by certain influences in the Church in the Sixth Century. The Second Council of Constantinople (A.D. 553) condemned it as a heresy, and from that time official Christianity frowned upon it, and drove it out by sword, stake and prison cell. The light was kept burning for many years, however, by that sect so persecuted by the Church—the Albigenses—who furnished hundreds of martyrs to the tyranny of the Church authorities, by reason of their clinging faith to the Inner Teachings of the Church concerning Reincarnation and Karma.

Smothered by the pall of superstition that descended like a dense cloud over Europe in the Middle Ages, the Truth has nevertheless survived, and, after many fitful attempts to again burst out into flame, has at last, in this glorious Twentieth Century, managed to again show forth its light and heat to the world, bringing back Christianity to the original conceptions of those glorious minds of the Early Church. Once more returned to its own, the Truth will move forward, brushing from its path all the petty objections and obstacles that held it captive for so many centuries.

Let us conclude this lesson with those inspiring words of the poet Wordsworth, whose soul rose to a perception of the Truth, in spite of the conventional restrictions placed upon him by his age and land.

> "Our birth is but a sleep and a forgetting,
>   The soul that rises with us, our life's star,
>   Hath elsewhere had its setting,
>   And cometh from afar.
>   Not in entire forgetfulness,
>   And not in utter nakedness,
>   But trailing clouds of glory do we come
>   From God, who is our home."

THE TWELFTH LESSON

THE MESSAGE OF THE MASTER

Running throughout nearly all of the teachings and messages of Jesus, is to be found the constant Mystic Message regarding the existence of the Spirit within the soul of each individual—that Something Within to which all can turn in time of pain and trouble—that Guide and Monitor which stands ever ready to counsel, advise and direct if one opens himself to the Voice.

"Seek ye first the Kingdom, and all things shall be added unto you." And, again, as if to explain: "The Kingdom of Heaven is within you." This is the Mystic Message which gives one a key to the Mysteries of the Inner Teachings.

Let us take up a few of His sayings and endeavor to interpret them by the light of these teachings. But before doing so we must call the attention of the student to the fact that, in order to understand intelligently what we are saying, he must carefully re-read the "Fourteen Lessons in Yogi Philosophy" wherein the details of the teachings are set forth—that is the fundamental truths are explained. In the "Advanced Course" and in "Gnani Yoga" the higher phases of the teachings are presented. And, although in the said works there is little or no reference made to Christianity, yet the teachings are so fundamental that the Inner Teachings of all religions—including Christianity—may be understood by one who has acquainted himself with these fundamental truths.

There is but one real Occult Philosophy, and we find it in evidence everywhere—once the Truth is grasped, it is found to be the Master Key with which to unlock the various doors leading to the esoteric phase of any and all religions or philosophies. The Yogi Fathers, centuries and centuries ago, solved the Riddle of the Universe, and the highest efforts of the human mind since that time have but corroborated, proven and exemplified the original Truth as voiced by these Venerable Sages.

Let us read the words of Jesus in the light of this Ancient Wisdom.

Let us consider the Sermon on the Mount as given in Matthew (Chapters 5; 6; 7).

"Blessed are the poor in spirit; for theirs is the Kingdom of Heaven." (Matt. 5:3.)

By these words Jesus indicated the occult teachings that those who renounced the vain glory and petty ambitions of this world would be on the road to the realization of the Real Self—the Something Within—the Spirit. For is it not written that "the Kingdom of Heaven is within you"?

"Blessed are they that mourn; for they shall be comforted." (Matt. 5:4.)

By these words Jesus pointed out the occult teachings that those who had so far advanced that they could see the folly of human ambition, and who consequently felt the pain that comes to all who stand above the crowd, and who mourned by reason of their realization of the folly and uselessness of all for which men strive so hard? would, in the end, be comforted by that "peace which passeth all understanding" which comes only to those who enter into a realization of the Kingdom of Heaven which is within them.

"Blessed are the meek; for they shall inherit the earth." (Matt. 5:5.)

By these words Jesus sought to teach that those who had acquired the attitude of obedience to the Power of the Spirit Within them would become as Masters of the things of earth. This message is frequently misunderstood by reason of the lack of perception of the Mystic meaning contained in the words. The word "meek" does not mean that "I'm so meek and humble" attitude and expression of the hypocritical followers of form. Jesus never taught this—and never acted it. He was always the Master, and never sought to make of his followers cringing creatures and whining and sniveling supplicants. He asserted His Mastery in many ways and accepted the respect due him—as for instance when the vial of precious ointment was poured upon Him. His use of the word, which has been poorly translated as "meek," was in the sense of a calm, dignified bearing toward the Power of the Spirit, and a reverent submission to its guidance—not a hypocritical and cowardly "meekness" toward other men. The assurance that such should "inherit the earth" means that they should become masters of things temporal—that is, that they should be able to rise above them—should become lords of the earth by reason of their "entering into the Kingdom of Heaven" within them.

"Blessed are they that hunger and thirst after righteousness; for they shall be filled." (Matt. 5:6.)

This is the promise of the Master that they who sought the Kingdom of Heaven (within them) should find it—that their spiritual hunger and thirst should be satisfied in the only way possible.

"Blessed are the merciful; for they shall obtain mercy." (Matt. 5:7.)

Here is taught the blessing for forbearance, kindness, tolerance and absence of bigotry, and the reward that comes as a natural consequence of such a mental attitude.

"Blessed are the pure in heart; for they shall see God." (Matt. 5:8.)

Here is the assurance that "to those who are pure all things are pure"—that the purity of one's own heart, and the recognition of the God Within, leads to a perception of the God within everything. "He who sees God within himself, sees Him in everything," says an old Persian writer. And verily such a one "sees God" where He abides—and that is Everywhere.

"Blessed are the peacemakers; for they shall be called sons of God." (Matt. 5:9.)

Here is the call to the disciple to use his wisdom and power in the direction of remedying the strife that arises from the differing conceptions of Deity and Truth prevailing among men. He who is able to point out the Truth underlying all religions and beliefs indeed becomes as a beloved son of God. He who is able to show that under all forms and ceremonies, under various names and titles, behind various creeds and dogmas, there is but one God, to whom all worship ascends—he is a Peacemaker and a Son of God.

> "Blessed are they that have been persecuted for righteousness' sake; for theirs is the kingdom of heaven. Blessed are ye when men shall reproach you, and persecute you, and say all manner of evil against you falsely for my sake. Rejoice and be exceeding glad; for great is your reward in heaven; for so persecuted they the prophets that were before you." (Matt. 5:10-12.)

In these words Jesus sought to comfort and encourage those who would be called upon to carry the Message in the centuries to follow. And one has but to look over the list of names of the courageous souls who have sought to keep the flame alight—to preserve the teachings in their original purity—to protect them from the cant, hypocrisy, self-seeking and formalism of those who sought and obtained places of power in the Church. The gibbet; the stake; the dungeon;—was their reward. But the Faith that was called into manifestation during the persecutions served to bring them to the realization of the Spirit, and thus indeed "theirs is the kingdom of heaven."

"But ye are the salt of the earth; but if the salt have lost its savor wherewith shall it be salted? It is henceforth good for nothing, but to be cast out and trodden under foot of men." (Matt. 5:13.)

Here Jesus warned against the failure of the Illumined to serve as the yeast which should leaven the mass of men by their thoughts and actions. The use of the term "salt" in this connection is familiar to all students of ancient mysticism. Food without salt was deemed unpalatable and undesirable. The Few were the salt of the earth, designed to render it worthy and perfect as a whole. But where a grain of salt had parted with its savor, there was naught else that could impart saltiness to it, and it became worthless and fit only for the refuse heap. The duty of the "salt" is to impart savor—the duty of the Elect is to impart savor to the race of men.

> "Ye are the light of the world. A city set on a hill cannot be hid. Neither do men light a lamp and put it under a bushel, but on the stand; and it shineth unto all that are in the house. Even so let your light shine before men; that they may see your good works, and glorify your Father who is in heaven." (Matt. 5:14-16.)

These words, like those preceding it, teach the Elect to shed abroad the light which has come to them. They are warned against concealing it beneath the cover of conventional conduct, but are urged to live and act so that men may perceive the light that is within them—the Light of the Spirit—and may see the right road by means of its rays. A man having the Light of the Spirit shining bright within him is able to rouse the lamps of understanding in the minds of other men, to become kindled and alight. That is the experience of the majority of those who read these words—they have had their lamps of knowledge kindled by the rays of the Spirit emanating from some soul, either by word of mouth, writings, or by personal contact. Spirituality is contagious! Therefore spread it! This is the meaning of this passage.

> "Think not that I came to destroy the law of the prophets: I came not to destroy, but to fulfill. For verily I say unto you, Till heaven and earth pass away, one jot or one tittle shall in no wise pass away from the law till all things be accomplished." (Matt. 5:17-18.)

In this passage Jesus asserted positively the fact that He was not teaching a new doctrine, but had come simply to carry on the work of those who had preceded Him. He asserted the validity of the Ancient Wisdom, and told that the Law that had been in force would so continue until heaven and earth should pass away—that is, until the end of this great World Cycle. In these words Jesus proclaimed His allegiance to the Occult Teachings. To those who would claim that He referred to the current Jewish teachings we would point out the fact that these he did come to destroy, for Christianity is opposed to the Jewish formalism and outer teachings. Jesus referred to the Inner Teachings, not to the outer religious creeds or forms. He came not to destroy the old Teachings, but merely to "fulfill," that is, to give a new impetus to the Ancient Wisdom.

> "Whoever therefore shall break one of these least commandments, and shall teach men so, shall be called least in the kingdom of heaven: but whosoever shall do and teach them, he shall be called great in the Kingdom of Heaven. For I say unto you, that except your righteousness shall exceed the righteousness of the scribes and Pharisees, ye shall in no wise enter into the kingdom of heaven." (Matt. 5:19-20.)

Here Jesus cautions against violating the fundamental occult teachings, or of teaching false doctrines. He also again bids men to do and preach the truth. Note the reference to the "kingdom of heaven." Again He points out that the "righteousness" required to gain the "kingdom of heaven" is a far different thing from the formalism, ceremonialism and "churchism" of the scribes and pharisees—people who, in that day, stood for that which the "churchy" preachers and their bigoted, narrow flock of sheep-like parishioners stand for today. It requires more than "faithful performance of church duties" to enter into the real "kingdom of heaven." Jesus was ever a foe of the narrow formalism which clings close to the empty forms and words, and which ignores the Spirit. Were He to return today, He would drive from the temples the horde of money-making preachers and hypocritical followers who make a mock of sacred things.

> "Ye have heard that it was said to them of old time, Thou shall not kill; and whosoever shall kill shall be in danger of the judgment: but I say unto you that every one who is angry with his brother shall be in danger of the judgment; and whosoever shall say to his brother 'Raca,' shall be in danger of the council; and whosoever shall say 'Thou fool' shall be in danger of the hell of fire. If therefore thou art offering thy gift at the altar, and there rememberest that thy brother hath aught against thee,

leave there thy gift before the altar, and go thy way, first be reconciled to thy brother and then come and offer thy gift. Agree with thine adversary quickly, while thou art with him; lest haply thine adversary deliver thee to the judge, and the judge deliver thee to the officer, and thou be cast into prison. Verily I say unto thee, Thou shalt by no means come out thence till thou hast paid the last farthing." (Matt. 5:21-26.)

These verses emphasize the teachings that sin consists not only of deeds and actions performed, but equally of thoughts and desires entertained and encouraged in the mind. The desire and thought, made welcome in the mind of a person, is the seed and germ of the sin or crime, even though they may never be manifested in action. To wish to kill is a sin, just as is the deed of killing. This is an old occult teaching, imparted to all candidates for Initiation.

"Ye have heard that it was said Thou shalt not commit adultery, but I say unto you that every one that looketh on a woman to lust after her hath committed adultery with her already in his heart. And if thy right eye causeth thee to stumble pluck it out and cast it from thee; for it is profitable for thee that one of thy members should perish and not thy whole body be cast into hell. And if thy right hand causeth thee to offend, cut it off and cast it from thee, for it is profitable for thee that one of thy members should perish and not thy whole body go into hell. It was said also, Whosoever shall put away his wife, let him give her a writing of divorcement, but I say unto you that every one that putteth away his wife, saving for the cause of fornication, maketh her an adulteress, and whosoever shall marry her when she is put away committeth adultery." (Matt. 5:27-32.)

In this passage, Jesus expressed the abhorrence of all advanced occultists for the abuse of the functions of sex. Not only the act, but the thought behind the act was condemned by him. The advanced occult teaching is that the function of the sex organization is entirely that of procreation—aught else is a perversion of nature. Jesus speaks in strong words to men and women, in this passage, regarding this great question. The concluding portion of the passage is a condemnation of the abuse of the marriage relation, and the privilege of divorce, which was being strongly agitated in His time.

He aimed a blow at the careless contracting of marriages, and the consequent careless dissolution of the tie. Jesus believed in the sacredness of the home life, and the welfare of the family. His utterance on this subject is unmistakably clear and forcible.

> "Again, ye have heard that it was said to them of old time, Thou shalt not forswear thyself, but shalt perform unto the Lord thine oaths: but I say unto you, Swear not at all; neither by the heaven, for it is the throne of God; nor by the earth, for it is the footstool of His feet; nor by Jerusalem, for it is the city of the great King; neither shall thou swear by thy head, for thou canst not make one hair white or black. But let your speech be Yea, yea, Nay, nay: for whatever is more than these is of the evil one." (Matt. 5:33-37.)

Here Jesus attacks the custom of swearing, which was so prevalent in His time among the Jews and other Oriental peoples. He urges simplicity and moderation of speech. In this He is true to the Occult traditions, which teach the value of simple thought and simple speech to all the Initiates and the Neophytes.

> "Ye have heard that it was said an eye for an eye and a tooth for a tooth, but I say unto you, Resist not him that is evil, but whosoever smiteth thee on thy right cheek, turn to him the other also, and if any man would go to law with thee and take away thy coat, let him have. And whosoever shall compel thee to go one mile, go with him two. Give to him that asketh thee and from him that would borrow of thee turn not away." (Matt. 5:38-42.)

In this passage Jesus alludes to the Law of Non-Resistance, which in its esoteric aspect is fully understood by all Initiates. This law is for application on the Mental Plane, and those who understand it, know that the precepts refer to the Mental Attitude of the Initiates toward others, which attitude is in itself a defense against imposition. Love turneth away Hate and Anger. The high thought neutralizes the evil designs of others.

> "Ye have heard that it was said Thou shall love thy neighbor and hate thine enemy. But I say unto you, Love your enemies and pray for them that persecute you, that ye may be sons of your Father who is in heaven, for he maketh

his sun to rise on the evil and the good, and sendeth rain on the just and the unjust. For if ye love them that love you, what reward have ye? Do not even the publicans the same? And if ye salute your brethren only, what do ye more than others? Do not even the Gentiles the same? Ye therefore shall be perfect as your heavenly Father is perfect." (Matt. 5:43-48.)

Here is taught that broad tolerance, charity and love that form such an important part of all of the mystic teachings. It is a doctrine entirely at variance with the orthodox idea of tolerance only to those who agree with one, or who may live in accordance with one's own views of life and conduct. It is the great broad doctrine of Human Brotherhood. Jesus teaches that God's love is bestowed upon all—the just and the unjust—and that this perfect love is the aim and goal of all who desire to attain to "the kingdom" of Spirit.

"Take heed that ye do not your righteousness before men, to be seen of them; else ye have no reward with your Father who is in heaven. When, therefore, thou doest alms sound not a trumpet before thee, as the hypocrites do in the synagogues and in the streets, that they may have glory of men. Verily I say unto you They have received their reward. But when thou doest alms let not thy left hand know what thy right hand doeth, that thine alms may be in secret and thy Father, who seeth in secret, shall recompense thee." (Matt. 6:1-4.)

This is another denunciation of ostentatious "churchiness" and "goodness," and religious posing. It is a lesson needed as much today as in the time of Jesus.

"And when ye pray, ye shall not be as the hypocrites, for they love to stand and pray in the synagogues and in the corners of the streets, that they may be seen of men. Verily I say unto you, They have received their reward. But thou, when thou prayest, enter into thine inner chamber, and having shut thy door, pray to thy Father, who is in secret, and thy Father, who seeth in secret, shall recompense thee. And in praying use not vain repetitions as the Gentiles do, for they think that they shall be heard for their much speaking. Be not therefore like unto them, for your Father knoweth what things ye have need of before ye ask him.

After this manner therefore pray ye: Our Father who art in heaven, Hallowed be thy name, Thy kingdom come, Thy will be done, as in heaven, so on earth. Give us this day our daily bread, And forgive us our debts, as we also have forgiven our debtors; And bring us not into temptation, but deliver us from the evil one. For if ye forgive men their trespasses, your heavenly Father will also forgive you. But if ye forgive not men their trespasses, neither will your Father forgive your trespasses." (Matt. 6:5-15.)

Here are the words of Jesus regarding the subject of Prayer. He cautions against the ostentatious exhibition of "piety," so prevalent in all churches, in all lands, in all times. He bids one approach the Father in a reverent spirit, devoid of all public notice. Then He gives to his disciples the famous "Lord's Prayer," in which is condensed a wealth of true religious instruction and precept. This glorious prayer needs no special interpretation. Let all students read the words themselves, filled with the realisation of the Spirit; and each will receive a message fitted to his requirements and development. The Lord's Prayer is a very Arcanum of the Mystic Message.

"Moreover, when ye fast, be not, as the hypocrites, of a sad countenance: for they disfigure their faces, that they may be seen of men to fast. Verily I say unto you, They have received their reward. But, thou, when thou fastest, anoint thy head and wash thy face, that thou be not seen of men to fast, but of thy Father, who is in secret, and thy Father, who seeth in secret, shall recompense thee." (Matt. 6:16-18.)

This is a caution against the "sanctimonious" attitude and pose assumed by certain "good" people of the churches, who would make a display of their adherence to and observance of forms. Jesus, as a true mystic, detested all religious posing and neglected no opportunities to condemn the same.

"Lay not up for yourselves treasures upon the earth, where moth and rust consume, and where thieves break through and steal: but lay up for yourselves treasures in heaven, where neither moth nor rust doth consume, and where thieves do not break through and steal: for where thy treasure is there will thy heart be also. The lamp of the body is the eye; if therefore thine eye be single, thy whole body shall be full of light. But if thine eye be evil, thy whole body shall be full of darkness! No man can serve two masters; for either he will hate the one and love the other, or else he will hold to one and despise the other. Ye cannot serve God and Mammon. Therefore I say unto you, Be not anxious for your life, what ye shall eat, or what ye shall drink; nor yet for your body, what ye shall put on. Is not the life more than the food, and the body than the raiment? Behold the birds of the heaven, that they sow not, neither do they reap, nor gather into barns; and your heavenly Father feedeth them. Are not ye of much more value than they? And which of you by being anxious can add one cubit unto the measure of his life? And why are ye anxious concerning raiment? Consider the lilies of the field, how they grow; they toil not, neither do they spin, yet I say unto you that even Solomon in all his glory was not arrayed like one of these. But if God so clothe the grass of the field, which today is, and tomorrow is cast into the oven, shall he not much more clothe you, ye of little faith? Be not therefore anxious, saying, What shall we eat? Or what shall we drink? Or wherewithal shall we be clothed? For after all these things do the Gentiles seek; for your heavenly Father knoweth that ye have need of all these things. But seek ye first then his kingdom, and his righteousness, and all these things shall be added unto you. Be not therefore anxious for the morrow; for the morrow will be anxious for itself. Sufficient unto the day is the evil thereof." (Matt. 6:19-34.)

This is the most remarkable passage in the New Testament. It is the most remarkable saying of Jesus of Nazareth. In it is condensed the whole of the occult teachings regarding the Conduct of Life. It condenses, in a few lines the entire doctrine of Karma Yoga—that branch of the Yogi Philosophy. It forms a veritable epitome of that which has been styled "The New Thought" as taught and expounded by its various cults and schools. There is no need of one reading and studying the various Metaphysical "Sciences" which have sprung into such favor of late years, if one will but read, ponder, study and practice the precepts of this wonderful passage of the Sermon on the Mount. Every sentence is a gem—a crystal of the highest mystic and occult philosophy. Book after book could be written on this one passage, and even then the subject would be but merely approached. The doctrine of single-mindedness toward the Spirit and the things of the Spirit, is taught. The folly of being tied to material things is pointed out. The lesson of non-attachment is forcibly put. But the great Truth expounded in this passage is the Power of FAITH. Faith is the Great Secret of all Occult Teachings and is the Key to its Inner Mysteries. Faith is the Master-Key that unlocks the doors of the Castle of Attainment. We trust that all students of these lessons will take this single passage from the Sermon on the Mount and memorize it. Make it a part of yourself—make it a part of your life—make it your rule of action and living. The life taught by this passage is the true life of the Spirit. Here is the true Light on the Path, for the guidance of the feet of all Mystics and Occultists!

> "Judge not, that ye be not judged. For with what judgment ye judge, ye shall be judged, and with what measure ye mete it shall be measured unto you. And why beholdest thou the mote that is in thy brother's eye, but considerest not the beam that is in thine own eye? Or how wilt thou say to thy brother, Let me cast out the mote out of thine eye, and lo, the beam is in thine own eye? Thou hypocrite, cast out first the beam out of thine own eye and then shalt thou see clearly to cast out the mote out of thy brother's eye." (Matt. 7:1-5.)

Here Jesus deals another powerful blow to the self-righteousness of the Pharisaical "good" people of the sects, creeds and cults of all lands, time and religions. He warns against that "Thank God! I am holier than thou" attitude that so many vain formalists affect in their dealings with other men. In these immortal words Jesus has sent ringing down the aeons of time a scathing rebuke to the hypocritical judges of other men—those men who wish to "reform" others to conform to their own standards. Out of the mouth of their Master are many so-called followers rebuked.

"Give not that which is holy unto the dogs, neither cast your pearls before the swine, lest haply they trample them under their feet and turn and rend you." (Matt. 7:6.)

Here is the warning to Initiates not to spread out a feast of their highest teachings to the mob, who with swinish instincts would defile the Divine Feast, and tear to pieces those who had spread it for them. The truth of this warning has been attested by the fate of those glorious souls who, disregarding it, attempted to give the Truth to the animal minds of the mob and were done to death for their folly. Even Jesus Himself met His fate from neglecting this very rule,—for allowing His sympathy to overcome His judgment.

"Ask and it shall be given you; seek and ye shall find; knock and it shall be opened unto you: for everyone that asketh receiveth, and he that seeketh findeth, and to him that knocketh it shall be opened. Or what man is there of you who if his son ask him for a loaf will give him a stone, or if he shall ask for a fish will give him a serpent? If ye then being evil know how to give good gifts unto your children, how much more shall your Father who is in heaven give good things to them that ask him? All things therefore whatsoever ye would that men should do unto you, even so do ye also unto them, for this is the law and the prophecy." (Matt. 7:7-12.)

Here is another burning message to men to live by the light of Faith in the Spirit. And a warning that unless one would act toward other men rightly, he could not expect to be dealt with rightly. It is the lesson of sowing and reaping—the lesson of the Law of Karma. Jesus is most emphatic in these statements. He does not alone say "Do this! Do that!" He states emphatically: "This is the Law!" And so it is—men are punished by their wrong deeds, not for them.

"Enter ye in by the narrow gate, for wide is the gate and broad is the way that leadeth to destruction, and many are they that enter in thereby. For narrow is the gate and straitened the way that leadeth unto life, and few are they that find it." (Matt. 7:13-14.)

This is the highest occult teaching. How few are they who find their way to the Realization of their own Divinity? Narrow indeed is the gate and straitened the way that leadeth to the goal. The masses follow the broad path, like fools—but few even see the narrow entrance to The Path.

"Beware of false prophets, who come to you in sheep's clothing, but inwardly are ravening wolves. By their fruits ye shall know them. Do men gather grapes of thorns, or figs of thistles? Even so every good tree bringeth forth good fruit; but the corrupt tree bringeth forth evil fruit. A good tree cannot bring forth evil fruit, neither can a corrupt tree bring forth good fruit. Every tree that bringeth not forth good fruit is hewn down and cast into the fire. Therefore by their fruits ye shall know them. Not every one that saith unto me, Lord, Lord, shall enter into the kingdom of heaven, but he that doeth the will of the Father who is in heaven. Many will say to me in that day, Lord, Lord, did we not prophesy by thy name, and by thy name cast out demons, and by thy name do many mighty works? And then will I profess unto them, I never knew you; depart from me, ye that work iniquity." (Matt. 7:15-23.)

Here is the notable warning against the perverted use of the occult powers—the prostitution of the Gifts of the Spirit—Black Magic, in short. For, as all well know, the occult forces may be applied to base as well as worthy uses. By their fruits shall ye know the good from the evil. He whose teachings render men weak, sheeplike and cringing, credulous leaners upon leaders, is a tree that bringeth forth evil fruit. Such are wolves in sheep's clothing, who fatten upon the bodies, substance and souls of their dupes. But those who lead men to be Men—yea, Super-Men—bring forth the good fruit of the Spirit. Be ye not deceived by names, words, creeds nor claims—nay, not even by miracles. Look always at the effect produced—the fruits of the tree—and govern yourself accordingly.

"Every one therefore that heareth these words of mine and doeth them shall be likened unto a wise man, who built his house upon the rock, and the rain descended and the floods came and the winds blew, and beat upon that house, and it fell not, for it was founded upon the rock. And every one that heareth these words of mine and doeth them not shall be likened unto a foolish man who built his house upon the sand, and the rain descended, and the floods came, and the winds blew and smote upon that house and it fell, and great was the fall thereof." (Matt. 7:24-27.)

In these parting words of the Sermon on the Mount Jesus gave a Message to all who would hear, or read His words, and profess to be His followers. He bade such build upon the eternal rock of the Truth—the rock of ages, that had its foundations in the very basic principles of Being. He warned them against building upon the shifting sands of theology and dogmatism, which would be surely swept away by the storms of Time. Upon the eternal Mystic Truths is Mystic Christianity founded. And it is still standing untouched by the storms of criticism, opposition and knowledge that have swept away many theological edifices in the past, and which are now beating with renewed vigor upon the remaining frail structures, which are even this day quivering under the strain.

Mystic Christianity invites the "New Theology," the "Higher Criticism," the "Criticism of Science"; for these will only tend to prove the truths of its fundamental principles. In Mystic Christianity, Religion, Philosophy and Science are known to be one and the same thing. There is no conflict between Science and Religion; Philosophy and Religion; or Philosophy and Science. They are all but names for the One Truth. There be but one Truth—there cannot be more than one. And so call it by the name of Religion—the name of Science, the name of Philosophy—it matters not, for the same thing is meant. There is naught but Truth—nothing else really exists. All that is not Truth is Illusion, Maya, Nothing. And Mystic Christianity is based upon the Rock of Truth, fearing not the winds nor the storms that try out the stability of all structures of thought. Like its founder, it has always existed—always will exist—from the Beginningless Beginning to the Endless Ending. The same yesterday, today, and tomorrow.

www.ingramcontent.com/pod-product-compliance
Lightning Source LLC
Chambersburg PA
CBHW011255040426
42453CB00015B/2412